With compliments

G. Pohl-Boskamp GmbH & Co. KG

Management and Control of Head Lice Infestations

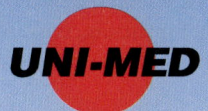

UNI-MED Verlag AG
Bremen - London - Boston

Heukelbach, Jörg:
Management and Control of Head Lice Infestations/Jörg Heukelbach.-
1st edition - Bremen: UNI-MED, 2010
(UNI-MED SCIENCE)
ISBN 978-3-8374-1203-1
ISBN 978-1-84815-154-3

© 2010   by UNI-MED Verlag AG, D-28323 Bremen,
              International Medical Publishers (London, Boston)
              Internet: www.uni-med.de, e-mail: info@uni-med.de

Printed in Europe

This work is subject to copyright. All rights are reserved, whether the whole or part of the material is concerned, specifically the rights of translation, reprinting, reuse of illustrations, recitation, broadcasting, reproduction on microfilm or in any other way and storage in data banks. Violations are liable for prosecution under the German Copyright Law.

The use of general descriptive names, registered names, trademarks, etc. in this publication does not imply, even in the absence of a specific statement, that such names are exempt from the relevant protective laws and regulations and therefore free for general use.

Product liability: The publishers cannot guarantee the accuracy of any information about the application of operative techniques and medications contained in this book. In every individual case the user must check such information by consulting the relevant literature.

MEDICINE - STATE OF THE ART

UNI-MED Verlag AG, one of the leading medical publishing companies in Germany, presents its highly successful series of scientific textbooks, covering all medical subjects. The authors are specialists in their fields and present the topics precisely, comprehensively, and with the facility of quick reference in mind. The books will be most useful for all doctors who wish to keep up to date with the latest developments in medicine.

Preface and acknowledgements

"Help! Lice alarm at school!"

Many parents, teachers, public health professionals, but also health care providers often are confronted with this situation, but not sufficiently prepared to manage it. Family members suffer from itching, teddy bears and helmets are put into freezers or sealed for weeks in plastic bags, curtains are vacuum-cleaned, all clothes and bed linen are washed, houses are desinfected, and children are kept out of school and not allowed to go to swimming pools.

The present book aims to clarify these and other common misconceptions regarding control of head lice. Written by leading experts in the field, scientific evidence on biology of lice, treatment, management and prevention options is discussed. A special focus is given on treatment options, the emergence of resistance to neurotoxic pediculicides, on new approaches to tackle this challenge, such as the use of silicone oils or spinosad, and on control measures in different settings. Topics rarely addressed when talking about head lice are covered, such as endosymbiotic bacteria as possible targets, oral treatments and the current knowledge regarding vaccination. Socio-cultural dimensions, knowledge of health professionals, and the possible role of lice as vectors for diseases have also been included.

Thus, I believe that this multi-faceted integrated approach, although presenting an old and common problem, will be of great value for all stakeholders involved—including parents, teachers, health care professionals, researchers and students. The book clearly cannot be a complete assessment of pediculosis, but is aimed to be a comprehensive paper, presenting up-to-date evidence.

I sincerely wish to thank all authors of this book who contributed with their outstanding competence. A special thank you to my family who so willingly contracted head lice for scientific purposes!

Fortaleza, Brazil, February 2010 *Jörg Heukelbach*

Authors

Gamal Elsayed Abou-Elghar, PhD
Department of Pesticides
Faculty of Agriculture
Menoufiya University
Shebin El-Kom MNF 32511
Egypt
aboelghar_gamal@hotmail.com

Chapter 6.5.

Liana Ariza, MPH
Department of Community Health
School of Medicine – Federal University of Ceará
Rua Prof. Costa Mendes 1608, 5. andar
Fortaleza CE 60430-140
Brazil
arizaliana@gmail.com

Chapter 5.2.

Sophie Bouvresse, MD
Department of Dermatology, Hôpital Henri Modor
51, avenue du Maréchal de Lattre de Tassigny
94010 Créteil
France
sbouvresse@hmn.aphp.fr

Chapters 6.2., 6.4.

Ian F. Burgess, BSc MSc MPhil FADO FRSH FRES
Medical Entomology Centre
Insect Research & Development Limited
6 Quy Court, Colliers Lane
Quy
Cambridge CB25 9AU
UK
ian@insectresearch.com

Chapters 2., 6.3., 6.12.

Craig G. Burkhart, MD MPH
University of Toledo College of Medicine
5600 Monroe Street, Suite 106B
Sylvania, Ohio 43560
USA
cgbakb@aol.com

Chapter 6.11.

Craig N. Burkhart, MD MSBS
Department of Dermatology
University of North Carolina at Chapel Hill
410 Market Street, Suite 400
Chapel Hill, NC 27516
USA
craig_unc@yahoo.com

Chapter 6.11.

Deon V. Canyon, PhD MPH FACTM AFAIM AFACHSE
Disaster Health and Crisis Management Unit
Anton Breinl Centre
James Cook University
Townsville, Qld 4811
Australia
deon.canyon@jcu.edu.au

Chapters 3.1., 6.7., 6.10., 7., 12.

Olivier Chosidow, MD PhD
Department of Dermatology, Hôpital Henri Modor
51, avenue du Maréchal de Lattre de Tassigny
94010 Créteil
France
olivier.chosidow@hmn.aphp.fr

Chapters 6.2., 6.4.

John Marshall Clark, PhD
Department of Veterinary & Animal Science
University of Massachusetts
Amherst, MA 01003
USA
jclark@vasci.umass.edu

Chapter 6.5.

Maria Danilevich, BSc
Department of Parasitology
Hebrew University-Hadassah Medical School
P.O. Box 12272
Jerusalem 91120
Israel
danilmar@yahoo.com

Chapter 8.

Hermann Feldmeier, MD PhD
Institute of Microbiology and Hygiene
Charité University Medicine, Campus Benjamin Franklin
Hindenburgdamm 20
12203 Berlin
Germany
hermann.feldmeier@charite.de

Chapters 1., 4., 5.1., 9.2., 11.

Leon Gilead, MD PhD
Department of Dermatology and Venereology
Hadassah Medical Center
P.O. Box 12000
Jerusalem 91120
Israel
leong@cc.huji.ac.il

Chapter 8.

Michaela Gorath, PhD
Medical Department
G. Pohl-Boskamp GmbH & Co. KG
Kieler Straße 11
25551 Hohenlockstedt
Germany
m.gorath@pohl-boskamp.de

Chapter 10.

Ulrich R. Hengge, MD MBA
Hautzentrum Prof. Hengge
Immermannstr. 10
40210 Düsseldorf
Germany
hengge@hautzentrum-hengge.de

Chapter 3.2.

Jörg Heukelbach, MD DTMPH MScIH PhD
Department of Community Health
School of Medicine – Federal University of Ceará
Rua Prof. Costa Mendes 1608, 5. Andar
Fortaleza CE 60430-140
Brazil

and

School of Public Health, Tropical Medicine and Rehabilitation Sciences
James Cook University
Townsville, Qld 4811
Australia
heukelbach@web.de

Chapters 1., 3.1., 3.2., 4., 5.1., 5.2., 6.6., 6.7., 6.8., 6.9., 6.13., 9.1., 9.2., 12.

Daniel Hilscher
Quality Assurance & Medical Devices
G. Pohl-Boskamp GmbH & Co. KG
Kieler Straße 11
25551 Hohenlockstedt
Germany
d.hilscher@pohl-boskamp.de

Chapter 10.

Arezki Izri, MD PhD
Department of Parasitology, Hôpital Avicenne
University of Paris 13
93009 Bobigny
France
arezki.izri@avc.aphp.fr

Chapters 6.2., 6.4.

Petra Kist, MDRA
Regulatory Affairs
G. Pohl-Boskamp GmbH & Co. KG
Kieler Straße 11
25551 Hohenlockstedt
Germany
p.kist@pohl-boskamp.de

Chapter 10.

Kim S. Larsen, PhD
KSL Consulting
Ramløsevej 25
3200 Helsinge
Denmark
kim@ksl.dk; www.ksl.dk

Chapter 6.1.

Si Hyeock Lee, PhD
Department of Agricultural Biotechnology
Seoul National University
Seoul 151-742
Republic of Korea
shlee@snu.ac.kr

Chapter 6.5.

Kosta Y. Mumcuoglu, PhD
Department of Parasitology
Hebrew University-Hadassah Medical School
P.O. Box 12272
Jerusalem 91120
Israel
kostam@cc.huji.ac.il

Chapter 8.

Michael Mumcuoglu, BA
Department of Parasitology
Hebrew University-Hadassah Medical School
P.O. Box 12272
Jerusalem 91120
Israel
xmichaelm@gmail.com

Chapter 8.

Fabiola A. Oliveira, MD MPH PhD
Gesundheitsamt
Beratungsstelle zu sexuell übertragbaren Erkrankungen einschl. AIDS
Neumarkt 15-21
50667 Köln
Germany
foliveira@web.de

Chapters 3.2., 6.6., 6.8., 6.9.

Julie Parison, B SocSc Hons
School of Public Health, Tropical Medicine and Rehabilitation Sciences
James Cook University
Townsville, Qld 4811
Australia
julie.parison@jcu.edu.au

Chapter 7.

Alberto Novaes Ramos Jr., MD MPH
Department of Community Health
School of Medicine – Federal University of Ceará
Rua Prof. Costa Mendes 1608, 5. Andar
Fortaleza CE 60430-140
Brazil
novaes@ufc.br

Chapters 5.2., 6.13.

Joachim Richter, MD DTM&H
Tropical Medicine Unit
University Hospital of Gastroenterology, Hepatology and Infectious Diseases
Heinrich-Heine-University
Moorenstr. 5
40225 Düsseldorf
Germany
Joachim.Richter@med.uni-duesseldorf.de

Chapters 3.2., 6.8.

Rick Speare, BVSc Hons MBBS PhD
School of Public Health, Tropical Medicine and Rehabilitation Sciences
James Cook University
Townsville, Qld 4811
Australia
richard.speare@jcu.edu.au

Chapters 3.1., 6.7., 6.13., 9.1., 12.

Win J. Tcheung, MD
University of North Carolina, Chapel Hill
2013 Pershing Street
Chapel Hill, NC 27705
USA
j.tcheung@gmail.com

Chapter 6.11.

Uade Samuel Ugbomoiko, PhD
Department of Zoology
Parasitology Unit
University of Ilorin
PMB 1515
Ilorin
Nigeria
samugbomoiko@yahoo.com

Chapters 3.2., 5.2.

Contents

1.	**Of Lice and Man—a Short History**	**18**
1.1.	References	21

2.	**Head Lice Biology**	**24**
2.1.	Morphology	25
2.2.	Feeding and water physiology	27
2.3.	Mating, eggs and reproduction	27
2.4.	Life cycle	29
2.5.	References	31

3.	**Epidemiology**	**34**
3.1.	Transmission and risk factors	34
3.1.1.	Fomite-to-head transmission	34
3.1.2.	Head-to-head transmission	37
3.1.3.	Social and behavioural transmission factors	37
3.1.4.	Risk factors	37
3.1.5.	Conclusions	38
3.1.6.	References	38
3.2.	Prevalence and incidence of head lice	40
3.2.1.	Prevalence	40
3.2.2.	Seasonal variation	40
3.2.3.	Incidence	41
3.2.4.	References	41

4.	**Clinical Aspects**	**44**
4.1.	Symptoms	44
4.2.	Signs	44
4.3.	References	45

5.	**Diagnosis and Rapid Assessment**	**48**
5.1.	Diagnosis of head lice infestations	48
5.1.1.	Diagnosis of active infestation	48
5.1.2.	Diagnosis of historical infestation	50
5.1.3.	References	50
5.2.	Rapid assessment of head lice infestations	51
5.2.1.	References	51

6.	**Treatment Options and Resistance**	**54**
6.1.	Mechanical removal of lice and eggs	54
6.1.1.	Lice and nit removal combs	54
6.1.2.	References	56
6.2.	Treatments using pediculicides with neurotoxic mode of action	56
6.2.1.	Natural pyrethrins and semi-synthetic pyrethroids	57
6.2.2.	Organophosphates (malathion)	57
6.2.3.	Other insecticides	57
6.2.4.	Formulations and application	58

6.2.5.	Adverse events and safety concerns	58
6.2.6.	Which insecticide should we choose?	59
6.2.7.	References	60
6.3.	Mechanisms of resistance	60
6.3.1.	References	63
6.4.	Resistance to chemical compounds	64
6.4.1.	Phenothrins	64
6.4.2.	Malathion	65
6.4.3.	Conclusions	65
6.4.4.	References	65
6.5.	Monitoring permethrin resistance in human head lice using knockdown resistance *(kdr)* gene mutations	66
6.5.1.	Molecular mechanisms of knockdown permethrin resistance	66
6.5.2.	Molecular detection of *kdr* mutations for resistance monitoring	67
6.5.3.	Determination of *kdr* allele frequencies in human head louse populations worldwide	69
6.5.4.	Head louse resistance management	71
6.5.5.	References	72
6.6.	Silicone oils for the treatment of head lice infestations	73
6.6.1.	References	76
6.7.	"Natural" treatments and home remedies	76
6.7.1.	Pyrethrins	77
6.7.2.	Tea tree	77
6.7.3.	Neem	78
6.7.4.	Quassia	78
6.7.5.	Ylang ylang	79
6.7.6.	Custard apple	79
6.7.7.	Clove	79
6.7.8.	Lippia species	79
6.7.9.	Coconut	80
6.7.10.	Vegetable oils	80
6.7.11.	Eucalyptus and other herbs	80
6.7.12.	Ovicides	80
6.7.13.	Conclusions	81
6.7.14.	References	81
6.8.	Oral drugs for the treatment of head lice	83
6.8.1.	Ivermectin	83
6.8.2.	Trimethoprim-sulfamethoxazole (co-trimoxazole)	84
6.8.3.	Albendazole	84
6.8.4.	Levamisole	85
6.8.5.	Phenylbutazon	85
6.8.6.	Thiabendazole	85
6.8.7.	References	85
6.9.	Other approaches for head lice management: spinosad and oxyphthirine®	86
6.9.1.	Spinosad	86
6.9.2.	Oxyphthirine®	87
6.9.3.	References	87
6.10.	Head lice repellents	87
6.10.1.	Repellent mechanisms	87
6.10.2.	Research on irritant-based tropotaxis	88
6.10.3.	Factors affecting efficacy and effectiveness	89
6.10.4.	Research on other repellent mechanisms	89

6.10.5.	Area repellents	90
6.10.6.	Lice repellents in humans	91
6.10.7.	Final considerations	92
6.10.8.	References	92
6.11.	Potential for future treatments targeting endosymbionts of head lice	93
6.11.1.	References	94
6.12.	Is immunisation the future of louse control?	95
6.12.1.	References	97
6.13.	General considerations on treatments and treatment schemes	97
6.13.1.	References	100

7. Head Lice and the Impact of Knowledge, Attitudes and Practices—a Social Science Overview — 104

7.1.	Knowledge	104
7.2.	Social attitudes about the infestation	104
7.3.	Practices	107
7.4.	Conclusion	108
7.5.	References	109

8. Knowledge and Practices of Health Professionals Regarding Head Lice — 112

8.1.	References	113

9. Prevention and Control — 116

9.1.	Control of head lice in developed market economies	116
9.1.1.	Prevention and health education	116
9.1.2.	Treatment	117
9.1.3.	Involvement of stakeholders	118
9.1.4.	The "No Nit Policy" and exclusion from school	118
9.1.5.	Conclusion	119
9.1.6.	References	119
9.2.	Control of head lice in resource-poor communities	120
9.2.1.	References	121

10. Regulatory Aspects of Head Lice Products — 124

10.1.	Medical devices	124
10.2.	Medicinal products	126
10.2.1.	Legal requirements	126
10.3.	Comment	128
10.4.	References	128

11. Lice as Vectors of Pathogenic Microorganisms — 132

11.1.	References	134

12. Internet Resources for Head Lice — 138

Index — 142

Of Lice and Man—a Short History

1. Of Lice and Man—a Short History

Sucking lice (*Anoplura*) are ectoparasites of mammals. The highly specialised blood-sucking insects complete their entire life cycle on the host. As mammalian blood differs widely among species in terms of suitability for louse nutrition, lice are usually host-specific. A paradigmatic example is the head louse *Pediculus capitis*, with humans as the only hosts.

Head lice have been parasitising humans since the emergence of our hominid ancestors. Given that the closest relative of the human louse is *P. schaeffi*, which infests chimpanzees, one might assume that human and chimpanzee lice have cospeciated with their hosts as family heirlooms, since they diverged from a common ancestor. This requires that the divergence among host and parasite approximates to the same timescale. However, whereas sucking lice of primates have undergone at least 25 million years of coevolution with their hosts, chimpanzee lice and human head/body lice last shared a common ancestor roughly 5.5 million years ago [1].

Phylogenetic analysis suggests that the louse genera *Pediculus* and *Pthirus* are each monophyletic and are sister taxa to one another [1, 2] (☞ Figure 1.1). The age of the most recent common ancestor of the two *Pediculus* species (the head louse and the body louse) matches the age predicted by host divergence, whereas the age of the ancestor of *Pthirus* does not [3]. This indicates that the divergence was contemporaneous with a split in cospeciation in the case of *Pediculus*, but not in the case of *Pthirus* [3]. The former event coincided with the divergence of ancestor primates into the lineage leading to chimpanzees and humans. Reed et al. [1] therefore suggested that the shared coevolutionary history of the anthropoid primates and their lice is a mixture of evolutionary events including cospeciation, parasite duplication, parasite extinction and host switching.

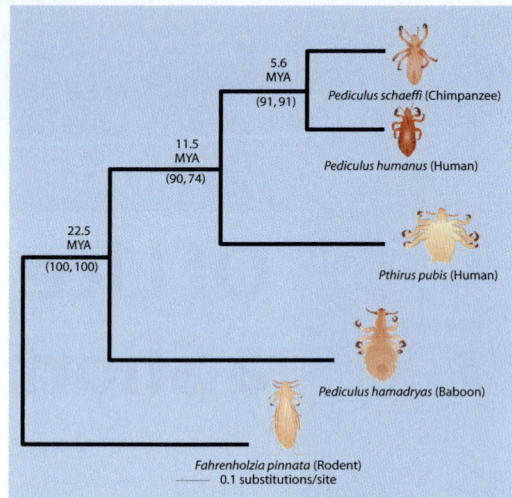

Figure 1.1: Phylogenetic tree of primate lice. Divergence dates are estimates from mitochondrial DNA data. Numbers in parentheses indicate bootstrap values (reproduced from Reed et al. [6]).

Mitochondrial DNA (mtDNA) studies have shown that there are three clearly divergent mitochondrial clades of *Pediculus* dating back up to 2 million years, each with a specific geographic distribution [4]. Mitochondrial genes, in contrast to other nuclear markers, do not show recombination and thus can be used to describe louse evolution. Therefore, the geographic distribution of mitochondrial clades provides clues on the evolution of lice and their human hosts.

The most common mtDNA is found among head and body lice (clade A) with a worldwide distribution. Recent mtDNA analysis of lice from pre-Colombian mummies indicates that their parasites belonged to clade A [5].

Clade B consists only of head lice and has been detected in the Americas, Europe and Australia, where it is the most prevalent louse lineage. A recent study provides evidence that the *living* population of clade B may have its origin in North America, but also that clade B ancestor lice originally did not arise in this region. There is reason to assume that this clade emerged in Africa together with its human ancestor host, and from there dispersed to other regions of the world and eventually reached the Americas (☞ Figure 1.2) [4]. Clades A and B were present in North America before the first Europeans arrived, and probably clade B lice migrated to Europe and Australia after the colonisation of the Americas and Australia (☞ Figure 1.2).

Clade C is most divergent clade and has been identified only among head lice from Nepal and Ethiopia [6].

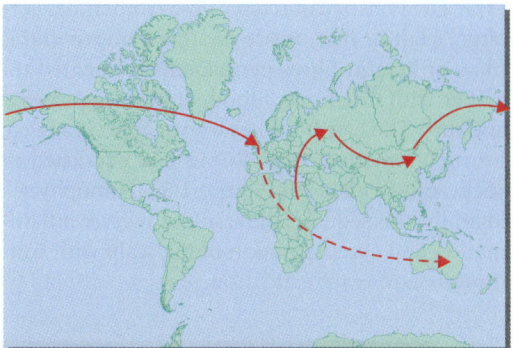

Figure 1.2: Putative migration routes of clade B head lice. These lice are believed to have migrated from Africa to Asia and subsequently to the Americas. During colonisation, Europeans would have taken clade B to Europe. Clade B was then introduced into Australia by European colonisation (adapted from Light et al. [4]).

How can humans harbour three clades of lice that apparently diverged from each other over a million years ago, when that separation is more than tenfold older than the emergence and dispersion of hominids from Africa? The answer is that the separation took place around the time of divergence of the ancestors of modern humans from *Homo erectus* [6]. At least two hominid lineages co-existed for about one million years until the demise of *H. erectus*, and there is some evidence that modern humans may have interbred with archaic humans. Even if interbreeding did not occur, they may well have exchanged their ectoparasites, for example, when *H. sapiens* encountered *H. neanderthalensis* in Europe roughly 100.000 years ago.

As lice have been infesting humans since the beginning of mankind, these and other ectoparasites are considered responsible for the loss of the dense layer of hair covering the body, a rather unusual finding among mammals [7, 8]. The loss of fur would have the evolutionary advantage of reduced loads of lice, fleas and other ectoparasites. Hairlessness would have been maintained by the naturally selected advantages in reducing diseases, and by sexually selected effects arising from mate choice for hairless partners, possibly in combination with other factors favouring hairlessness [7].

Clearly, loss of fur has its disadvantages, such as increased exposure to sun, heat loss at low temperatures and less protection from physical injury—if the hominid ancestors had retained their fur, they surely would have been better protected from cold nights and daily sunshine [8]. Thus, the loss of a dense layer of thick fur has only been possible when humans developed intelligent means to cover their body with leather and textiles, to control fire and to produce shelters, allowing a flexible response to changing temperatures. This may also be the reason why monkeys maintained their fur during evolution.

Lice and nits have been found in 8.000 to 10.000 years old textiles, hairs and combs excavated from archaeological sites such as on the Aleutian Islands, in South West USA, Mexico, Peru and Brazil, as well as in Egyptian mummies [9, 10] (☞ Figure 1.3). In ancient times, pediculosis capitis occurred independent of social classes—remains of head lice have been identified in the hair of noble persons buried in Egypt 3.000 years ago, in nomad Indians of North America, as well as in subsistence farmers in Greenland. In Southern Peru, prevalence of head lice infestation in prehistoric mummies varied between 18% and 71%, according to the archaeological site, and was higher in males than females, probably because men more commonly had braids [10]. In fact, for much of human prehistory and history head and body lice have been so prevalent and were so closely linked to everyday human life that they became part of the language. For example, we speak about feeling lousy and admonish our friends for nit-picking. In Germany hard times are called *"lausige Zeiten"* (lousy times) and little rascals of the neighbourhood considered *"Lausebengel"* (lousy boys).

In the 16th, 17th and 18th centuries head lice infestations were very common in all classes of society in Europe (☞ Figure 1.4). During that period most of aristocracy and gentry shaved their hair and wore wigs. Some have suggested that this custom had arisen to protect the bearer of the wig from lice. However, historical anecdotes are not in line with this assumption. For instance, the English naval administrator and Member of Parliament Samuel Pepys (1633-1703) complained in his diary more than once about his wig being infested with head lice: *"Thanks to my barbers, to have my periwig cleared of its nits."*

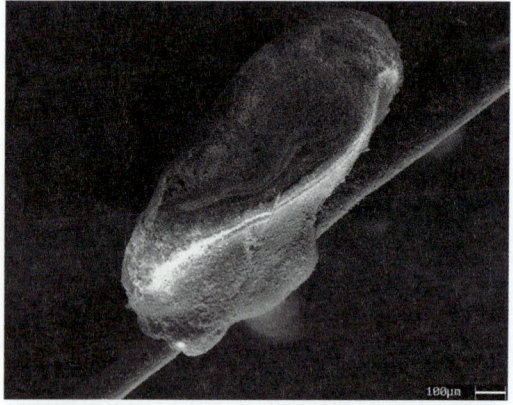

Figure 1.3: A 10.000 year-old nit attached to a human hair from an archaeological site in northeast Brazil (image kindly provided by Prof. Adauto Araújo, Rio de Janeiro, Brazil).

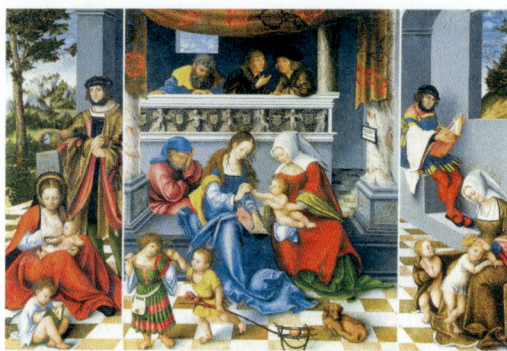

Figure 1.4: Renaissance painting of Lucas Cranach der Ältere (1472-1552) entitled *"Tryptichon mit der Heiligen Sippe"* (Tryptichon with the Holy Kinship), also known as the *"Torgauer Altar"* (1509). It shows the Holy Kinship (extended family of Jesus descended from his grandmother St. Anne). In the centre, three generations including grandmother St. Anne, her daughter Virgin Mary and Jesus can be seen. On the right side, Mary's sister Salome is passing a head lice comb on her son, the apostle James. The relaxed facial expression of mother and child indicate that this procedure used to be common in the 16th century, when the painting was made. Original at Städelmuseum, Frankfurt (Germany).

In the 19th century head lice infestations remained extremely common mainly in lower social classes, such as in poor urban neighbourhoods of big cities, where workers and their families lived crowded under precarious conditions. The inhabitants of the dwellings were infested by all kind of ectoparasites, including head and body lice [11].

A sequel of persistent heavy head lice infestation is known by the name of Polish plait (*Plica polonica*) [12]. The Polish plait is typically a (sometimes very large) plait of hair, made of a hard impenetrable mass of keratin fibres permanently cemented together with dried pus, blood, old lice egg-casings and dirt. The hair becomes irreversibly entangled, forming a matted, malodorous and encrusted or sticky moist mass (☞ Figure 1.5). Pathophysiologically, this sequel is the result of a severe inflammation and eczematisation of the scalp with continuous exuberant exudation.

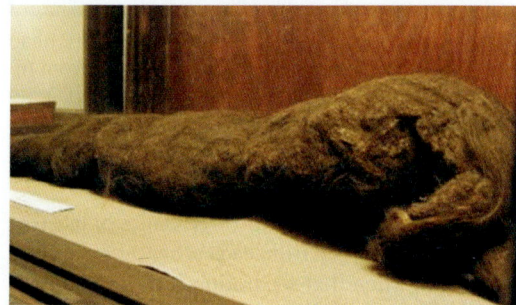

Figure 1.5: A 1.5-meter long Polish plait kept in the History of Medicine Museum in Krakow, Poland.

The Polish plait was quite common in the 17th, 18th and 19th centuries, but Reinhard & Buikstra [10] also identified a monstrous plait in a 1000 year-old mummy of the Chiribaya Culture in Peru. The Polish plait affected mostly the peasantry, but was not unusual also among higher social classes [12]. One of the most notable persons in history said to be afflicted was King Christian IV of Denmark (1577-1648). His plait had the form of a pigtail hanging from the left side of his head, adorned with a red ribbon.

The British diarist Hester Thrale (1741-1821) described in her book *"Observations and reflections made in the course of a journey through France, Italy and Germany"* a Polish plait she saw in the collection of the Elector of Saxony in Dresden in 1786: *"…the size and weight of it was enormous, its length four yards and a half (about 4 m). The person who was killed by its growth was a Polish lady of quality well known in King Augustus's court."*

In the second half of the 19th century in the Ukraine, Professor Józef Dietl made a particular effort to eradicate Polish plaits. He organised an official census of people suffering from the disease —which rapidly spawned rumours that plaits would be taxed. The fear to have to pay tax was said to have helped eradicate the Polish plait in the region—an interesting example of cost-effective morbidity control.

1.1. References

1. Reed DL, Light JE, Allen JM, Kirchman JJ. Pair of lice lost or parasites regained: the evolutionary history anthropoid primate lice. BMC Biol 2007;5:7.

2. Light et al. What's in a name: The taxonomic status of human head and body lice. Mol Phylogenet Evol 2008; 47:1203-1216.

3. Weiss RA. Apes, lice and prehistory. J Biol 2009;8:20.

4. Light et al. 2008. Geographic distributions and origins of human head lice *(Pediculus humanus capitis)* based on mitochondrial data. J Parasitol 2008;94:1275-1281.

5. Raoult D, Reed DL, Dittmar K, Kirchman JJ, Rolain JM, Guillen S et al. Molecular identification of lice from Pre-columbian mummies. J Infect Dis 2008;197:535-543.

6. Reed DL, Smith VS, Hammond SL, Rogers AR, Clayton DH. Genetic analysis of lice supports direct contact between modern and archaic humans. PLoS Biol 2004; 2:e340.

7. Pagel M, Bodmer W. A naked ape would have fewer parasites. Proc R Soc Lond B 2003 (Suppl.) 270:117-119.

8. Rantala MJ. Human nakedness: adaptation against ectoparasites? Int J Parasitol 1999;29:1987-1989.

9. Araujo A, Ferreira LF, Guidon N, Maues Da Serra FN, Reinhard KJ, Dittmar K. Ten thousand years of head lice infection. Parasitol Today 2000;7:269.

10. Reinhard & Buikstra 2003. Louse Infestation of the Chiribaya Culture, Southern Peru: Variation in Prevalence by Age and Sex. Mem Inst Oswaldo Cruz 2003;98 (Suppl. I):173-179.

11. Evans RJ. Tod in Hamburg: Stadt, Gesellschaft und Politik in den Cholera-Jahren 1830-1910. Rowohlt, Reinbek, Germany, 1990.

12. Narbutt SO. Über den Weichselzopf plica polonica. Medizinische Fakultät zu München, 1879.

Head Lice Biology

2. Head Lice Biology

Head lice are obligate, blood feeding, parasitic insects found only on the heads of humans. As sucking lice they are classified as belonging to the Sub-Order Anoplura of the Order Phthiraptera, a group restricted to mammals. *Homo sapiens* is unusual among anthropoids in having lice from two genera, *Pediculus* (☞ Figures 2.1 and 2.2) and *Pthirus* (☞ Figure 2.3), each occupying different bodily habitats and, in the case of *Pediculus* being divided into two more or less distinct behavioural and ecological forms, head lice and clothing/body lice, that may or may not be from a single species. Table 2.1 shows currently recognised species from these two genera.

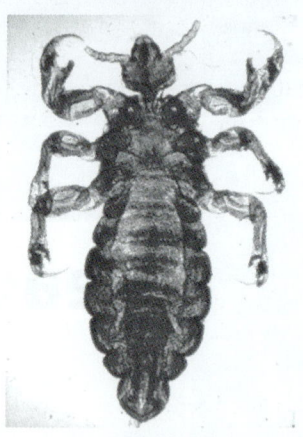

Figure 2.2: Body (clothing) louse adult male.

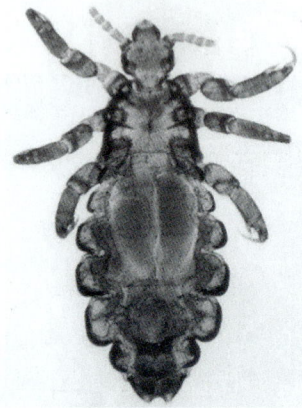

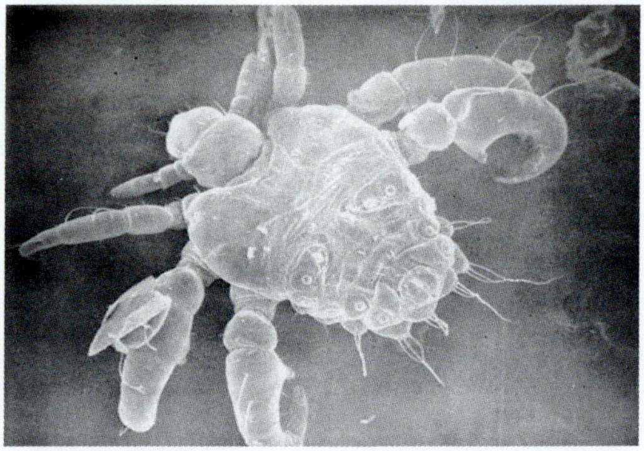

Figure 2.1: Head louse adult female.

Figure 2.3: *Pthirus pubis*, the crab louse or pubic louse.

Morphologically, human lice have physical differences (☞ Figures 2.1-2.3), for example, head lice are normally smaller and more likely to have deep lateral insections between the segments of the abdomen (☞ Figure 2.1), whereas clothing lice tend to be larger and have only slight indentations where the segments meet (☞ Figure 2.2). How-

Family of lice	Genus of lice	Species of louse	Host genus
Pediculidae	*Pediculus*	*humanus*	*Homo* (human)
		capitis	*Homo* (human)
		schaeffi	*Pan* (chimpanzee)
		mjöbergi	*Ateles* (spider monkey)
Pthiridae	*Pthirus*	*pubis*	*Homo* (human)
		gorillae	*Gorilla* (gorilla)

Table 2.1: Species of lice infesting humans and other anthropoids.

ever, these features are not consistent between or even within populations even from the same host, but using other less variable characteristics, such as the length of the tibial and tarsal segments of the second pair of legs, did allow separation of lice from these double infestations into distinct populations that correlated with their distribution on the host [1]. On this basis Busvine (1978) concluded that the two ecological forms were separate species that did not interbreed, and this conclusion was also drawn by evaluation of genetic markers that demonstrated head and clothing lice from the same host were genetically distinct, that is head lice remained on heads and clothing lice remained on clothing [1, 2].

In parallel it has been shown that head lice and clothing lice in one geographical region may be more closely related to each other than the head lice are related to head lice from another region, suggesting they are conspecific [3].

This also appears to confirm the suggestion that clothing lice are simply head lice that migrated from heads and took up residence in clothing, a feature that may occasionally be seen in children who have heavily infested heads and change their clothing infrequently. However, under normal circumstances head lice are negatively geotropic, which can be easily demonstrated by transferring a head louse onto the clothing and watching it rapidly climb back up to the scalp. Consequently, it is still not clear whether head lice should be referred to as *Pediculus capitis*, a distinct species [1, 2], or *P. humanus capitis* [3] but as the former allows a clear distinction, and due to the overriding ecological separation currently found in nature that probably eliminates the risk of current and future interbreeding for most populations, which ultimately will lead to a clear separation, in this book we refer to them as *P. capitis*.

2.1. Morphology

A description of the appearance and structure of *Pediculus* lice was described by Buxton (1947) in his monograph on lice [4]. Adult head lice are more or less elongate, with a distinct head, a short fused thorax, and an oval shaped, clearly segmented abdomen with seven visible segments (☞ Figures 2.1 and 2.4). The head has a pair of five segmented antennae and a pair of eyes that each consists of a single ocellus. As with other blood feeding insects the mouthparts are modified to form long needle like stylets but in the case of sucking lice they are fully retracted into the head when not in use but everted by muscular action when the mouth is applied to the skin of the host in order to feed. The louse maintains its position against the skin during feeding by means of a ring of teeth on the haustellum that are pushed out with the stylets and grasp the stratum corneum of the host (☞ Figure 2.5).

The midgut is large and extends from the mid thorax for most of the length of the abdomen and when replete fills up to 30% of the abdominal space. It is constantly moving with peristaltic activity and freshly ingested blood mixes with remains of previous blood meals still held in the midgut. At intervals, a small quantity of the fluid content passes from the midgut into the hindgut and passes rapidly to the anus where it appears as a droplet that immediately coalesces to form a more or less dry and solid pellet of faecal matter [4].

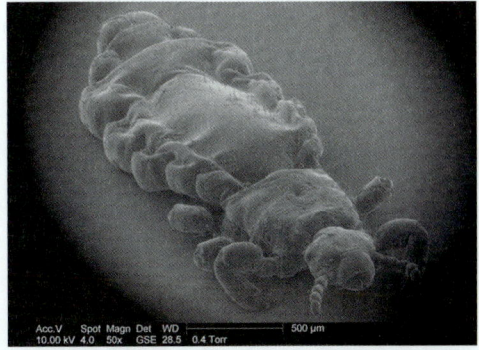

Figure 2.4: Head louse showing deep indentations at the margins of seven visible abdominal segments.

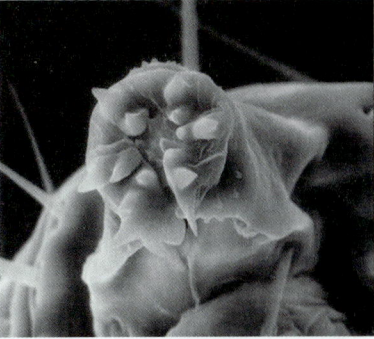

Figure 2.5: Haustellum partially elevated showing buccal teeth.

The thorax is highly sclerotised and appears to have a central hole, the notal pit, which is actually the external base for a hollow rod used for fixation of the muscles that operate the legs. The legs are robust and short and have highly modified segments suited to living amongst the hairs. The most distinctive of these are the tibiae, which carry a thumb-like extension on the tip of the ventral side. This "thumb" opposes with a mobile claw that articulates with the apex of the single tarsal segment (☞ Figure 2.6). The space formed between the claw and the thumb is able to enclose and grip almost all human head hairs, irrespective of whether they are rounded, oval, or flattened in cross section.

The thorax also carries a single pair of spiracles on the protonum. These have a collar or peritreme around the nearly circular opening, which leads into a flask shaped chamber lined with a complex matrix of plates and ridges forming a honeycomb complex around the sides [7]. This in turn passes through a glandular mass, the spiracular gland before joining with the tracheal system. The abdominal spiracles are smaller but have a more complex internal structure. They are mounted along the sides of the abdomen on large, sclerotised paratergal plates.

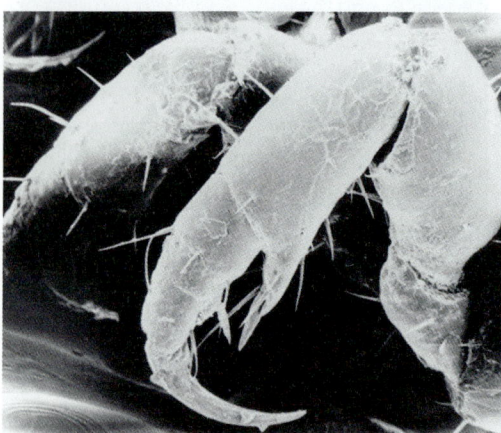

Figure 2.6: Leg and claw of *Pediculus*.

Most of the abdomen has a membranous cuticle through which can be seen some internal structures, including the gut filled with blood, the so-called mycetome organ that contains symbiotic micro-organisms, tracheae filled with air, and sometimes other organs outlined against the dark gut contents, including eggs developing in the oviducts of females. The gut opens in a sub-terminal anus, which is close to but separate from the genital opening. The tip of the abdomen is rounded in males but often appears pointed because the tip of the statumen penis, which can be seen through the cuticle on the underside as a chestnut coloured pair of rods joined at the tip, protrudes through the genital opening (☞ Figure 2.7).

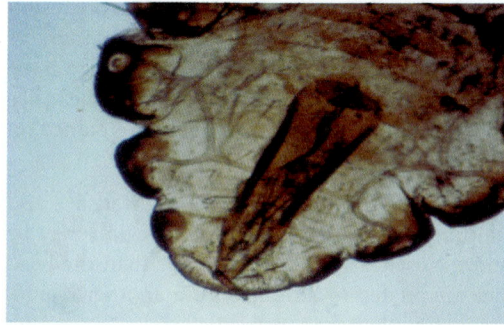

Figure 2.7: Head louse terminalia showing statumen penis.

The female abdomen has a v-shaped notch at the tip that is formed by a pair of lobes and on the underside there is distinctive pigmented shield-shaped plate in front of the genital opening and a pair of smaller lobes called gonopods, which are used to align the egg during laying (☞ Figure 2.8).

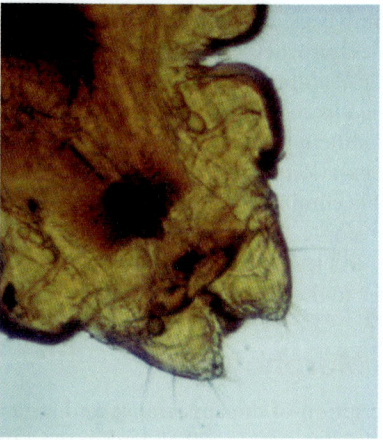

Figure 2.8: Head louse female terminalia showing gonopods.

2.2. Feeding and water physiology

Head lice need to feed relatively frequently and so must remain on their host continuously. When the louse feeds it attaches to the host skin and probes until it pierces a suitable blood vessel after which it injects saliva into the wound to prevent the blood from clotting as it sucks up the mixture of fluids. As the cuticle of the louse is partially transparent blood can be seen as a thread of blood passing through the head, under a low power microscope, as it is pumped from the mouth to the midgut. The blood is moved rapidly by two small muscular pumps, the cibarial and pharyngeal pumps in the head, which appear to flicker as they fill with blood and expel it.

It is not clear how often head lice must take blood but, lice fed at 6 hour intervals died after a few days [5] and it has been suggested that around six or more blood meals each day are necessary for most head lice [6]. Head lice removed from their host may remain active in a relatively cool and moist atmosphere for more than a day without feeding. If replaced on the host within a few hours they may be able to feed and re-establish. However, between about three and 18 hours after removal from the host they become incapable of drawing blood, presumably because they are too dehydrated to produce enough saliva to prevent the blood from clotting.

This occurs because they have an unusual water physiology. Most blood feeding insects excrete excess water taken in as part of their food either as urine or as liquid faeces. Sucking lice produce dry faeces that minimises faecal contamination of the host skin and hair, which could alert the host to their presence. As an alternative strategy for water management they excrete water by transpiration through the respiratory system. This is unusual because most small insects employ extensive strategies to conserve water and is a contradiction of Buxton's assertion that water vapour loss is minimised by contraction of the tracheal occlusor muscle to constrict the trachea, a process that could also prevent inflow of fluid when a louse is immersed in water. However, Webb [7] noted that the occlusor is more likely to cause the duct between the spiracle and the trachea to gape, opening rather than closing the aperture, which could increase the rate of water loss. Additional water loss could be of benefit soon after feeding, when the abdomen of the louse is distended with fluid, but it appears the mechanism cannot be switched off so unfed lice quickly become non-viable.

2.3. Mating, eggs and reproduction

Adult lice mate soon after completion of their final moult, although females do not normally begin to lay eggs until they have been adult for at least 24 hours. Male lice attempt to mate with most lice of an appropriate size. This means they may approach adult females, other males, or even well developed third stage nymphs. The initial approach is made by the male pushing his head and body beneath the potential mate from behind the tip of the abdomen. Once underneath the other louse he raises the tip of his abdomen and probes the tip of the abdomen of the potential mate. If the other louse is a receptive female she lowers the tip of the abdomen and the male grasps her second or third pair of legs using the claws of his first pair of legs, which are larger than the claws found on the second and third legs. Mating begins by insertion of the mesomere and the partially fused parameres of the aedeagus into the female genital opening in order to dilate it. This dilatory device is then reflexed to one side and the remainder of the aedeagus is inserted. The functional part of the aedeagus, the endophallus, consists of two main parts the statumen or true penis and the vesica penis, an inflatable sac covered with spine like protrusions that lock with the roughened surface of the inside of the vagina. Copulation is relatively prolonged, sometimes taking 30 minutes or more, and both participants must contribute to the separation process, so if one dies during the mating process the other is unable to separate them.

The females lay only one egg at a time because each is so large that it occupies up to 20% of the abdominal volume. There are two ovaries that produce an egg alternately and egg production continues even if the female has not been mated or if the sperm from a previous mating have degenerated or been used up. Therefore, lice mate with some regularity and frequency to ensure continued fertility and male lice move continuously in search of fresh mates. When a female louse is well fed and laying eggs at maximum capacity it may be possible to see one complete egg ready for laying through the translucent cuticle, one well developed partially formed egg in the other ovary, and occasionally the beginnings of a third egg in the same ovary as the fully formed egg.

Egg laying is a relatively rapid process. The females fix their eggs to hairs close to the scalp using a secretion from accessory glands opening into the oviduct. The louse first locates a suitable place on the hair, and then strokes it using the gonopods, perhaps to check that it is free from dust and debris or else to ensure the correct alignment for the egg. She then extrudes a droplet of the fixing secretion followed rapidly by the egg, laid base first into the droplet. At the same time the louse moves forward to deposit the egg and to ensure she is not stuck to the hair because the secretion hardens rapidly forming a cylindrical tube on that part of the hair and a cup like coating to the base of the egg. The fixative material is extremely resilient and holds the eggshell in place long after the embryo has emerged (☞ Figure 2.9). However, the fixative is not a chemical "glue" but rather it is formed from peptide molecules that contract during the setting process so the cylinder surrounding the hair shaft grips it to prevent the egg from sliding.

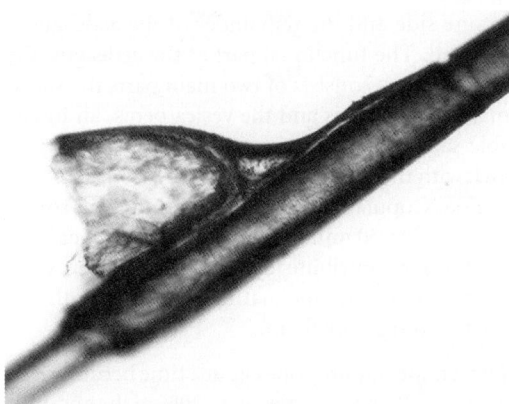

Figure 2.9: Abraded nit.

The egg of the head louse is approximately ovoid in shape and 888 ± 27 microns long by 460 ± 22 microns wide [8]. The more pointed end is laid into the fixative and the wider end has an oval opening sealed in life by a cap that fits into a reflexed rim. The cap is dome shaped and is thickened to form a double layer pierced by 7-11 pores or aeropyles that open into a chamber within the cap, which in turn opens into the inside of the eggshell via a complex microcapillary (☞ Figure 2.10). The eggshell is more or less transparent and encloses a tough chorionic membrane that surrounds the developing embryo and protects it from dehydration and chemical action.

It is unclear how many eggs a louse lays each day because reports based on small numbers of insects maintained in artificial containers vary considerably. In general the rate at which a female head louse lays eggs increases sharply over the first few days, is maintained at a peak rate for about two weeks and then steadily declines until the louse dies [9]. The average number of eggs laid daily was found to be around 4.9 ± 0.2 eggs per day from four geographically distinct populations from the Americas. This is a much lower fecundity than may be found in some popular literature, which is often based on estimated extrapolations from results obtained with clothing lice rather than experiment and observation of head lice. In the same study the mean longevity for female head lice was 20.2 ± 1.4 days (range 12 to 31), which means that even if a louse were to be capable of laying eggs at maximum rate throughout her life she would only be able to produce about 100 eggs in total. However, not all eggs are fertilised and even those that are do not always hatch. The hatch rate from these experiments was approximately 77% and fertility declines as the females age.

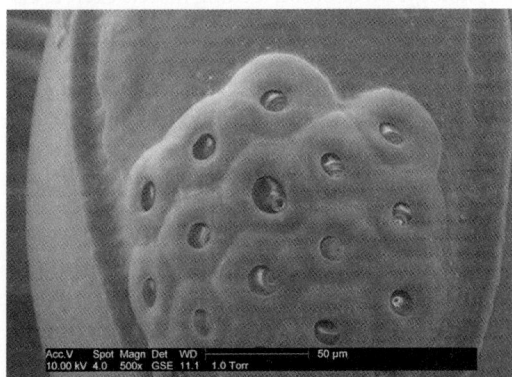

Figure 2.10: Louse egg aeropyles showing the opening of the inner microcapillary tubule.

As head louse eggs are placed on the hairs close to the scalp, this provides adequate warmth for optimum development. A high proportion of eggs are laid on hairs behind a line that runs from the tips of the ears to the top of the crown of the head. This region has more closely spaced hairs, irrespective of how dense or sparse the hairs are overall, which not only maintains a more stable temperature close to the scalp but also retains humidity more effectively so there is less risk for dehydration of the developing embryo.

There are no published data for the time taken for development of head louse eggs at scalp temperatures. Although Takano-Lee recorded fecundity and longevity *ex vivo* the eggs were incubated at a lower temperature (29° ± 1° Celsius) than scalp temperature (between 34° and 36° Celsius depending upon position on the head and the individual concerned). Similarly, figures given by Buxton [4] (taken from Leeson) are not for development rates of head louse eggs but of clothing louse eggs, although these are often quoted, and misquoted. The only experimental data in the public domain for head louse eggs maintained at body temperature are those of Lang (a PhD thesis). He found that at 36° ± 2° C eggs hatched in 5-6 days, which interestingly is consistent with the clothing louse figures of hatch in 5-7 days at 35° C and 7-9 days at 32° C given by Buxton [4].

The newly laid head louse egg is mainly colourless and translucent but may appear pigmented because it acts like a lens to focus the colour of the surrounding hairs. As it develops, firstly clusters of cells can be seen, which then coalesce to form the outline of a developing louse. The so-called "eyespot" is the first distinguishable characteristic, which normally appears during the third to fifth day of development, as a pinkish spot and darkens to black over the following day or two (☞ Figure 2.11). Near to the time of emergence the legs and claws can be seen, with distinguishable brownish claws. When the embryo is fully developed, the louse nymph pierces the chorionic membrane with its egg teeth and sucks air into its gut. Bubbles of air can be seen passing through the gut and being expelled from the anus. This causes a pressure increase in the shell behind the insect which then is pushed forward to release the cap of the eggshell, after which it pushes and pulls itself out. Some of the chorionic membrane is normally dragged out from within the shell as the nymph emerges. The empty shell, known as a nit, remains fixed to the hair for weeks or months, and due to refraction of light from the inner surface of the shell appears whitish in colour and is easily detected with the naked eye, whereas an embryonated egg is difficult to distinguish from its surroundings.

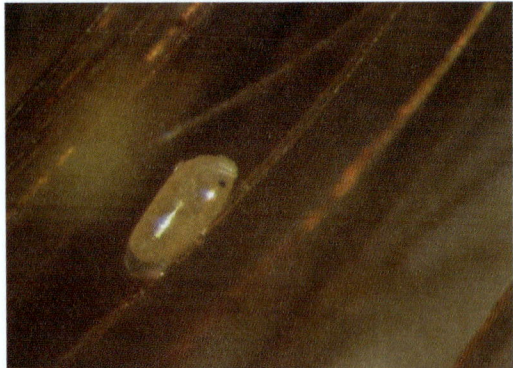

Figure 2.11: Head louse egg showing the eyespot of the developing embryo.

2.4. Life cycle

The newly emerged first instar nymph feeds soon after emergence, following which it appears red from the ingested blood. Subsequent meals do not make the body appear as bright red due to mixing with partially digested blood. The development of the nymphal head louse through three instars lasts approximately 9 days (☞ Figure 2.12), with each instar approximately the same length, although some individuals and populations may vary slightly [9].

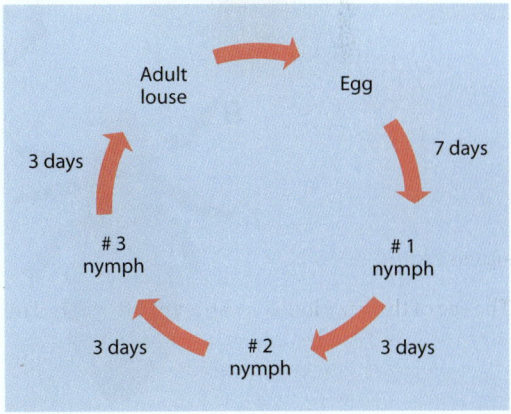

Figure 2.12: Diagram of the life cycle of the head louse.

Physically nymphs appear similar to adults apart from smaller size, a relatively smaller and less well defined segmentation of the abdomen, and no external sexual differentiation (☞ Figure 2.13). During the third instar, the symbiotic micro-organisms from the mycetomes of female nymphs migrate to the spongy walls of the oviduct, from where they can enter developing eggs when the louse becomes adult. Eggs that do not have symbiotes fail to develop, and if the mycetome is removed surgically or the symbiotes killed by antibiotic action nymphs cannot complete their development and die (details ☞ Chapter 6.11.).

Head lice, when not feeding, mating or laying eggs, pass most of the time in a relatively inactive state. Most life stages hold onto hairs with the claws on all their legs, align their bodies with the hair shafts with their heads pointing towards the scalp. This position allows the lice to move backwards and forwards along the hair shafts with ease. They can walk just as well backwards as forwards. Head lice can also move transversely across a bundle of hairs. To do this they do not rotate to stand at right angles to the hairs and walk forwards, rather they step sideways, maintaining their alignment with the hairs, moving their claws from one hair shaft to another in the manner of a crab walking. This has an advantage for avoiding detection because the body of all head lice has some pigment, which varies in quantity depending upon the origin, darker lice being found in geographic regions where the skin and hair of the hosts is darker and paler in regions where predominantly fair-haired and skinned people occur. Contrary to the suggestion from Buxton that the pigment of the louse is acquired during the first days of life in response to the darkness of its background, pigmented cuticle in lice is inherited, as can be seen from lice maintained in laboratory colonies, which may demonstrate several colour variants that persist over numerous generations despite being maintained under identical conditions. There is also a common misconception in the general population that head lice

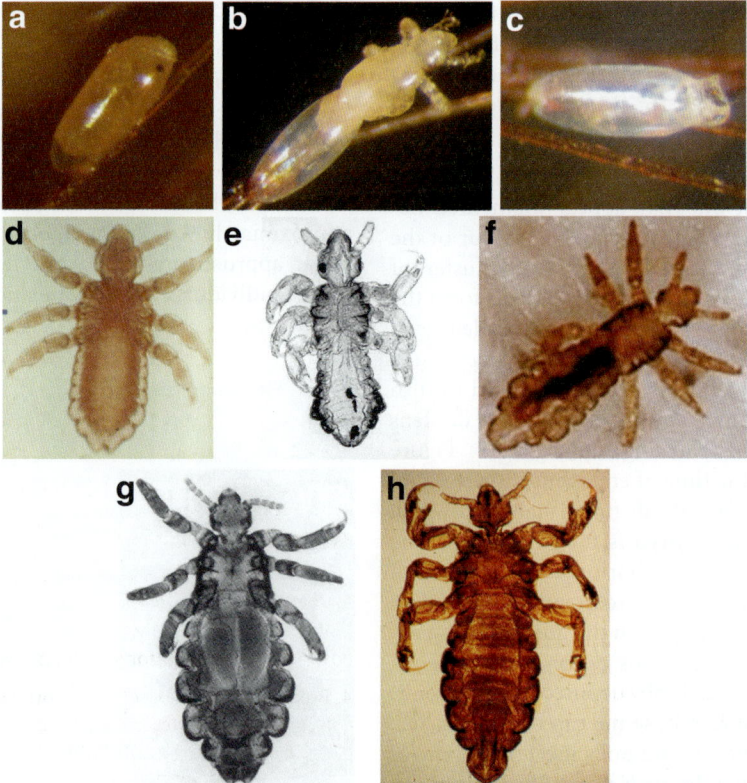

Figure 2.13: Life cycle stages of human lice. **a:** Egg with embryo; **b:** Nymph emerging from egg; **c:** Empty eggshell (nit); **d:** First stage nymph; **e:** Second stage nymph; **f:** Third stage nymph; **g:** Adult female; **h:** Adult male.

change their colour according to the environment —with the naked eye paler head lice simply look darker after blood feeding.

Pigmented cuticle in head lice occurs along the sides of the thorax, on the paratergal plates, and the claws in all lice. Additionally the males may have pigmented bands of cuticle across each segment of the abdomen. The intensity and depth of colour and the breadth of each of these pigmented zones is the primary colour variation so that lice may appear almost colourless through to nearly black. In addition the partially digested blood in the gut provides an additional dark stripe along most of the length of the body. As a result most lice appear to have three longitudinal stripes of colour, which when aligned with the hairs blends in with the background in much the same way that the striped camouflage on tigers and zebras breaks up their outline to make them less detectable in their habitat. As a result examining hair with head lice hiding amongst it makes finding them difficult. Consequently, the predominance of different pigment forms in lice in any particular community or ethnic group is mainly due to elimination of those insects that are more readily detected. Thus pale lice are easily seen and eliminated by people "nit-picking" in cultures where people have darker skins and hair and, similarly, dark lice are more easily identified and removed when contrasted against pale skin or hair.

Head lice have a series of proprio-receptors in their legs that warn the insect of any disturbance of the hair such as the host scratching or brushing or combing. Contrary to popular belief that head lice "move rapidly away" from disturbance of the hair, for which there is no evidence, it is, however, likely that insects aligned with the hair shafts may move closer to the scalp or simply cling more closely to the bundle of hairs. Consequently, even a search with a comb may fail to detect a louse. However, if the hair is then left undisturbed for a short time the louse may begin to move again and may be found quite easily with a comb.

Host transfer is initiated by disturbance of the hair, which stimulates lice in the appropriate physiological state to respond by moving towards the outer layers of the hair. First and second stage nymphs are less active than older stages and more inclined to remain close to the scalp. This means they are less likely to transfer to another host. However, when nymphs reach the third instar of development they become more mobile and, like young adults, may transfer to a new host. This dispersal behaviour is similar to most other organisms that migrate in search of mates and suitable breeding sites as they reach sexual maturity. It appears the males are the most mobile, presumably because they are constantly seeking females, as a result it is not uncommon for the first louse to invade a head to be a male.

The adult life span of a head louse is probably determined more by risks in the environment than other factors. Lice maintained under the sheltered conditions of culture containers, fixed to the arm of a volunteer in the laboratory, averaged around 20 days for both males and females, with a maximum of 32 days [9]. However, in the wild most head lice are likely to die sooner as a result of host activity such as scratching, grooming, or hair washing, each of which may injure or displace the insect. Consequently, it appears that head lice survive mainly because their hosts are unaware of their presence and because they do not cause their hosts significant harm rather than through high fecundity and any adaptations to avoid detection by running away. Head lice are beautifully adapted to their environment and exploit it efficiently, which is why they have survived for thousands of years, despite the efforts of humans to eradicate them.

2.5. References

1. Busvine JR. Evidence from double infestations for the specific status of human head lice and body lice (Anoplura). Syst Entomol 1978;3:1-8.

2. Leo NP, Hughes JM, Yang X, Poudel SKS, Brogdon WG, Barker SC. The head and body lice of humans are genetically distinct (Insecta: Phthiraptera, Pediculidae): evidence from double infestations. Heredity 2005;95:34-40.

3. Leo NP, Campbell NJH, Yang X, Mumcuoglu K, Barker SC. Evidence from mitochondrial DNA that head lice and body lice of humans (Phthiraptera: Pediculidae) are conspecific. J Med Entomol 2002;39: 662-666.

4. Buxton PA. The Louse: An Account of the Lice Which Infest Man, their Medical Importance and Control, 2nd edn. 1947, Edward Arnold & Co.: London.

5. Burgess IF, Brown CM, Peock S, Kaufman J. Head lice resistant to pyrethroid insecticides in Britain. BMJ 1995; 311:752.

6. Maunder JW. The appreciation of lice. Proceedings of the Royal Institution of Great Britain 1983;55:1-31.

7. Webb JE. Spiracle structure as a guide to the phylogenetic relationships of the Anoplura (biting and sucking lice), with notes on the affinities of the mammalian hosts. Proceedings of the Zoological Society 1946;116:49-119.

8. Kadosaka T, Kaneko K. Studies on sucking lice (Anoplura) in Japan (Part 6). A comparative observation of human lice eggs. Jap J Med Entomol Zoology 1985;36: 343-348.

9. Takano-Lee M, Yoon KS, Edman JD, Mullens BA, Clark JM. *In vivo* and *in vitro* rearing of *Pediculus humanus capitis* (Anoplura: Pediculidae). J Med Entomol 2003;40:628-635.

Epidemiology

3. Epidemiology

3.1. Transmission and risk factors

It can be tempting to examine the global spread of pediculosis in terms of transmission risks because most countries have experienced increases in the detection of *Pediculus capitis* since the 1900s [1]. Reducing transmission is arguably the most important factor controlling the spread of infestations [2]. However, the spread of emergent and resurgent diseases due to increased population movement is well documented and pediculosis is no exception. Of far more importance is the issue of reinfestation, which is a common problem in the control of pediculosis. Reinfestation is a highly problematic social and economic transmission issue that even effective pediculicides cannot easily resolve.

This chapter considers factors that have a bearing on the transmission of head lice. This has not been a clear-cut topic and there has been difficulty in estimating the importance of head-to-head versus fomite-to-head transmission. This has resulted in some time being invested during the last decade to determine the mechanisms involved in *P. capitis* transmission so that control programs do not squander limited resources [3]. Some of these studies are field-based while others involve laboratory experimentation under controlled conditions. As can be expected, results from these two sources do not always agree.

The lack of evidence and proliferation of unsubstantiated myths have resulted in epidemiological studies in different countries speculating on the primary mode of transmission with varying conclusions [4-10]. While *in vitro* studies continue to demonstrate that fomite transmission is possible, the body of field evidence concludes that head-to-head transmission is the primary mechanism and several likely fomite candidates have been shown to be inconsequential.

3.1.1. Fomite-to-head transmission

In 1993, it was stated that head lice *"willingly transfer from one host to another in the same species by the slightest bodily contact"* [3]. It was proposed that transmission may take place during head-to-head contact, but also when:

- Hairs carrying crawling forms of lice are dislodged from a louse-infested person and are deposited onto the head or body of an uninfested person.
- Lice are blown off an infested head onto an uninfested person.
- Lice are expelled through static charge from an infested head onto an uninfested person (e.g. during combing).
- Lice that have been separated from a person and which are moving on various fomites come into contact with an uninfested person [3].

Factors relating to head-to-fomite transmission and fomite-to-head transmission are both relevant here. One factor of key importance is that fomite-to-head transmission relies on the capacity of a louse to survive off-host long enough to come into contact with a new host. Body lice may live up to 10 days off a host at 15°C, 5 days at 24°C and 3 days at 30°C [11]. Early studies on head lice found them to quickly perish from starvation when removed from a host. Lice survived 9-11 hours at 25-37°C in low humidity and 10-14 hours in higher humidity, but survived up to 44 hours at 15°C in higher humidity [5, 12]. A more recent study confirmed that most lice were dead 40 hours post-blood meal [13]. The exact impact of these data and how they influence transmission rates from one substrate to another whether living or inanimate, have not yet been determined. In addition, fully active lice usually do not leave the head without any reason. Lice leaving the head may be close to dying, and it can be assumed that a high fraction of lice found on fomites are not capable of infesting a person.

While the survival rates of lice on fomites may be low, it is possible that gravid females could lay eggs that could later hatch and infest other hosts. Questions arising from this are: Do lice on fomites really lay eggs? If yes, what are the survival and hatch rates of fomite-laid eggs? *In vivo*-reared lice eggs take 8.4 days (range 6-11) to hatch with a hatch rate of 76%. However, when eggs are exposed to a human for 8 hours each night they take 15.2 days to hatch and only 58-59% hatch [14, 15]. There are no available

3.1. Transmission and risk factors

data for survival rates of eggs in unfavourable off-host circumstances, but one may assume that the egg hatch rates on fomites is low.

In a series of novel experiments on head lice placed on hair in an experimental laboratory setting, it was demonstrated that all lice encountering a blast of hot air from a hair dryer were dislodged [14]. Combing was also responsible for dislodging 100% of lice from hair in this setting. Towelling removed 60% and around 30% passively transferred from the hair to an alternative substrate. It was concluded that *"louse transmission by fomites may occur more frequently than is commonly believed and at close proximity may suffice to increase the likelihood of a new infestation."* However, we have encountered numerous anecdotal accounts of infested persons using hair-dryers and combs and they were never 100% free of lice. Nor did infested people reduce their lice populations by 60% each night as they towelled their hair. So laboratory results are often not in congruence with reality.

The advice of fomite-to-head advocates is to launder *"everything within the infested individual's bed... and thorough vacuuming of floors, carpets, and upholstery with a standard vacuum cleaner, or otherwise cleaning"* [14]. From the evidence-base, it is clear that fomite-to-head transmission is possible, but is unreasonably supported by some researchers to be sufficiently important to warrant cleaning of an infested person's environment [2]. As we have seen thus far and as we will see as more evidence is presented, this advocacy is not based on sound conclusions, has not been demonstrated to be effective in the field and places an unwarranted burden on already overburdened households.

Head lice researchers at the Anton Breinl Centre for Public Health and Tropical Medicine (ABC), James Cook University, Townsville (Australia) looked at several questions relating to the role of the environment in transmission of head lice in primary school. Their major, evidence-based, transmission-related findings related to the presence of lice on school hats, school floors and pillow slips of infested children. Hats have always been considered high-risk items. The general public and even many head lice researchers are of the opinion that hats and other apparel worn by infested people harbour lice. For instance: *"Fomite transmission is common with pediculosis capitis. The source of transfer is often headwear, shared hats, brushes, combs, earphones, bedding, upholstered furniture, and rugs"* [3]. To test the validity of this assertion, in the ABC study over 1000 hats in four schools were investigated for lice [16]. No head lice were found in all these hats and over 5500 head lice were captured from the heads of surveyed students. In another unpublished study conducted in a different primary school, a further 1000 hats were examined for lice. A single louse was identified on a hat belonging to a student whose hair had just been treated one hour earlier. It was assumed that this was a louse not killed by the treatment and was exhibiting the flee response [3]. This empirical data demonstrated that the odds of head lice transmission via hats of lice-infested children is sufficiently low to be considered improbable and inconsequential.

An epidemiological study on New York schoolchildren investigated the sharing of lockers and wall hooks for clothing and headwear as a risk factor for pediculosis. Although an association was found, a replication of this study in Pennsylvania schools found no association [4].

As such, transmission via articles of personal clothing appears to be a well-established myth. When considering why it is so entrenched, one can only speculate that it originated from older generations more familiar with body lice which prefer to reside in host clothing.

Another common recommendation by many companies, web sites and articles in the popular press is to treat and clean rugs, carpeting or floors when an infestation is found. The recommendation appears to be based on the belief that head lice can survive in the environment of the home or school and that people can be infested from this environment. However, no data exist in the scientific literature to support this contention. Transmission of head lice from floors to people makes little evolutionary or biological sense, but the lack of data to quantify this potential route of transmission means recommendations cannot be evidence-based. This idea was put to the test by ABC researchers who carefully vacuumed the floors of 118 primary school classrooms and searched the contents for any signs of head lice [17]. A median of only 1.6 g of vacuum debris was obtained from each classroom prior to evening cleaning by school janitors taking place. No lice or eggs were found in any of this debris, but all samples contained parts of insects or occasionally whole insects. Ants and parts thereof were the most commonly identified insects found. This was notable because of the amount of lice found on the heads of children in these classrooms: 466 students out of the total of 2230 children examined from the 118 classrooms had head lice, a prevalence of 21%. A rather staggering total of 14033 lice were captured from the infested students and mean intensity of infestation of 30.1 (21.9-38.3, 95% CI) lice per infested child and a median intensity of 6 lice were calculated. Of the infested students, 58% had less than 10 lice, 35% had 10-99 lice, 8% had 100-499 lice, and one 4-year-old girl preschooler had 1623 lice. One hundred and eight of the 118 classrooms (91.5%) had at least one infested student with active pediculosis and an average of 130 lice per infested classroom was calculated. Thus, the idea that lice transmission takes place from floors to people is a fictitious myth that has been debunked. The risk of acquiring head lice from the floors of school classrooms is zero and for the control of head lice there is no benefit in any activities to remove head lice from floors.

As already discussed, advice abounds on what to wash and clean if you have a head lice infestation, but the evidence for these assertions is anecdotal or laboratory-based and very little, if any, in the way of supporting field evidence is ever presented to back up these claims. At the heart of the matter are a number of questions about healthy active head lice:

- How often do they become dislodged from their host?
- What do they do when they find themselves on a fomite?
- Do lice on fomites constitute a significant transmission problem?
- Do they actively leave their hosts to wait on fomites for a chance occurrence with another host?
- Do they intentionally traverse fomites to cross from one host to another?

To develop an evidence base from which start addressing some of these questions, researchers at the ABC investigated the proportion of head lice populations found on pillow cases of people with head lice, and tested strategies to kill head lice on pillow cases [15]. To assess the occurrence of head lice on pillow cases, people with active pediculosis had their head lice collected and counted and the pillow case they had used the night before examined for head lice. To test strategies to kill head lice on pillow cases, live head lice were experimentally placed in miniature pillow cases, and the cases subjected to a hot wash, a cold wash, hot dryer, and hanging out to dry on an outdoor clothes line. In this study, 48 infested participants were recruited who were found to be harbouring 1845 head lice. The mean and median intensity of infestation was high: 38.4 and 21 lice, respectively. Of the 48 pillow cases, two cases had a single live nymph present and a third had a single dehydrated nymph. Thus, the occurrence of overnight live lice transference to pillow cases was 4.2% and proportionately, 0.1% of the head lice population actively transferred onto a fomite. The second part of the study found that heat (hot wash and hot clothes dryer) killed head lice experimentally placed in pillow cases while cold wash and hanging pillow cases out to dry did not kill head lice.

To add another dimension, one of the authors was once travelling in remote Aboriginal communities in northern Australia and happened one night to sleep in a "men's house" with 5 other men. The author slept on the left of the group with his head approximately 2 feet away from the next person's head and at no time was his head in contact with the next person's head. Nevertheless, the author found himself infested the following day. No other body contact was made before or after this event, which could have resulted in transmission. Lice thus will most certainly cross fomites to get from one host to another if the distance is small. Other studies have found that family size, overcrowding and sleeping in the same bed in fact can promote transmission [18-22]. The only conclusions that can be drawn from this study and experience are that pillow cases do pose a slight risk for transmission or reinfestation but that risk is low enough to be considered unimportant compared to other modes of transmission. However, if other potential hosts are around, this mode of transmission becomes far more likely and important. Changing and washing pillow cases in a situation where multiple infested and uninfested people are cohabiting is thus a waste of resources and time.

Three epidemiologic studies have demonstrated that there is no association between head lice presence and the sharing of combs and brushes, and one found an association [9, 23, 24]. In the latter study, which took place in Canada, no lice were found on the brushes of 10 children with active pediculosis [24]. The body of evidence thus suggests that this mode of transmission is possible, but most likely of little consequence compared to other modes.

3.1.2. Head-to-head transmission

The main route of transmission appears to be by head to head contact, but this is occasionally debated [3, 16], because there is limited experimental evidence and only indirect field evidence. However, as noted previously in this chapter, the role of other modes of transmission is more controversial and often has no substantial evidence-base.

Official advice for control of head lice frequently include recommendations to treat bedding, soft toys, clothes and to clean the household environment [25]. Head lice found on furnishings have been proposed as dead, sick, senile or injured [26]. One author noted active head lice on pillows in Bangladesh [27].

Findings in Australia have shown that infestations in urban primary schools are hyper-endemic with the main source of infestation identified at the classroom level [28]. If fomites were a significant contributor to this transmission, lice would have been found in school hats and on classroom floors. Since lice were not found in these environments, the clustering of pediculosis cases within classrooms can only implicate close contact as the primary mode of transmission variable.

In 2001, a laboratory study was published on spatial and kinetic factors of head lice transmission [29]. This study demonstrated that hair-to-hair transfer is strongly influenced by spatial and kinetic factors. For instance, lice found it easier to transfer if passing hairs moved slower; if hairs passed by them from toe to head; if hairs passed over their lateral surface; and if hairs passed parallel to the orientation of a louse. Optimum transferral only occurred when all these conditions were present. The relatively low overall transfer proportion of 7.1% in ideal circumstances did not support the assertion that transmission takes place between individuals *"by the slightest bodily contact"*, as discussed above [3].

3.1.3. Social and behavioural transmission factors

The physical and mechanical aspects of head lice transmission indicate that they are of minor importance. Transmission from fomites ranged from zero to 0.1% probability while transmission from hair to hair only occurs 7.1% of the time. So, what other factors have a significant impact on continuing high infestation rates? In 2006, the ABC head lice research team recognised that social and behavioural factors were extremely important. They designed a simple study and collected data through their website (www.jcu.edu.au/school/phtm/PHTM/hlice/hlinfo1.htm) from people suffering from head lice infestation. The study suggested that sociological and behavioural factors could decrease the effectiveness of control strategies (☞ Chapter 7. for details).

Another recent unpublished study by the authors investigated student and parent reactions to head lice infestations using a questionnaire approach. Fifty-three percent of respondents did not care that they had lice and 70% of these were males. A third of White students (36%) and only 17% of Asian students evinced negative emotion to being infested. The dominant parent reaction upon finding out that their child was infested was to immediately treat the condition. However, 14% of parents showed no reaction or response. The number of students who did not know they had lice was very high: female 60%, male 40%, Whites 45%, Asians 65%. While Asian students all informed their parents when they became aware that they were infested, 15% of White students concealed their infestation from their parents to avoid annoying them, to avoid anger or to avoid treatment.

3.1.4. Risk factors

Race and country of residence are not risk factors for infestation, as Gratz said in the 1997 WHO report, *"The head louse persists almost everywhere as the most common human ectoparasite"* [1]. However, in particular locations, there are racial variations due to the lice having physiologically adapted to the "native" population and being less suited to take advantage of more recent human populations [27].

In countries that attempt to resolve pediculosis, infestations are more common in primary schoolchildren, but all age groups are susceptible to head lice infestation [27, 28, 30].

Head lice can also be a problem in the elderly which may indicate an immunological susceptibility [31]. On the remote island of Satawal, Micronesia, the author found that pediculosis is viewed as socially desirable and infestation is encouraged with the result that most of the population is infested. When the group of most active social groomers were asked if anyone did not have lice, they were able to identify 10 women who could not support head lice even when lice were repeatedly placed on their heads. The reason for this is likely to be immunological which suggests that some people may be more susceptible than others. This is supported by another observed extreme where a young girl consistently was found to be harbouring over a 1000 lice whenever inspections by the ABC head lice team took place.

Gender was reviewed by Burgess in 1995 who found it to be of limited significance, if any [27]. Some studies found slightly more females with lice, but this was attributed to female behaviour being more social rather than any genetic or physiological factor. Two studies found gender to be a risk factor independent of hair length [28, 32]. In the author's recent unpublished study, the 136 high school participants all had a history of head lice and gender was not an apparent risk factor with 53.8% males and 46.2% females. However, in other socio-cultural settings, gender differences may occur [33]. The results for gender are conflicting and further research is required to clarify the gender effect.

Aspects of hair are anecdotally commonly related to head lice infestation, but this is not supported by conclusive data. Some studies have found a correlation between hair length and infestation while others have not [9, 19, 34, 35]. In an Israeli study, boys with medium length hair and girls with short hair experienced the most lice infestation [30]. The same study reported that brown and red hair were infested more than black or blond hair. In the author's recent unpublished study, hair thickness varied (thin 17.4%, medium 49.2%, thick 33.3%), colour varied (blond 16.7%, brown 67%, black 16.7%), and length varied (short 45.7%, shoulder length 27.9%, long 26.4%). These factors were not different from the uninfested population, so aspects of hair did not constitute obvious risk factors.

Since the ability to wash clothes is a socio-economic factor, hygiene was easily recognised as a risk factor for body lice, but this is not true for head lice, which do not reside in clothing. Quite to the contrary, an inverse relationship was found between pediculosis and socioeconomic status and researchers have found that washing hair only produces cleaner lice [9, 26, 36, 37].

3.1.5. Conclusions

A comprehensive awareness of the biology and ecology of *Pediculus capitis* and the epidemiology of pediculosis leads to the conclusion that fomite-to-head transmission occurs, but that it is relatively unimportant. The emergence of data on transmission factors over the past decade has definitively enabled head lice researchers to state that head-to-head transmission is the major route. However, transmission is a product of several inter-related variables, and physical factors pale into insignificance when compared to social and behavioural factors. The degree of apathy and neglect so clearly stated by students about themselves and their parents is the primary reason why control programs do not work, even if a highly efficacious pediculicide is used that is not affected by resistance of head lice.

Thus, the control of head lice should focus on the head, not on the environment, and schools and other institutions wishing to be proactive should invest their resources into educational approaches if they wish to render their mass treatment campaigns more effective.

3.1.6. References

1. Gratz NG. Human lice: their prevalence, control and resistance to insecticides: a review 1985-1997. Geneva: World Health Organization, Division of Control of Tropical Diseases, WHO Pesticide Evaluation Scheme; 1997.

2. Burkhart CN, Burkhart CG. Fomite transmission in head lice. J Am Acad Dermatol 2007;56:1044-1047.

3. Burkhart CN, Burkhart CG. The route of head lice transmission needs enlightenment for proper epidemiologic evaluations. Int J Dermatol [Letter]. 2000;39:878-879.

4. Juranek DD. *Pediculus capitis* in school children. In: Orkin M, Maibach H, editors. Cutaneous infestations and insect bites. New York City1985. p. 199-211.

5. Nuttall GHF. The biology of *Pediculus humanus*. Parasitology 1917;10:80-185.

6. Mellanby K. Natural population of the head-louse (*Pediculus humanus capitis*: Anoplura) on infected children in England. Parasitology 1943;34:180-183.

7. Slonka G, McKinley T, McCroan J, Sinclair S, Schultz M, Hicks F, et al. Epidemiology of an outbreak of head lice in Georgia. Am J Trop Med Hyg. 1976; 25: 739-743.

8. Sinniah B, Sinniah D, Rajeswari B. Epidemiology of *Pediculus humanus capitis* infestation in Malaysian school children. Am J Trop Med Hyg 1981;30:734-738.

9. Mumcuoglu K, Miller J, Gofin R, Adler B, Ben-Ishai F, Almog R, et al. Head lice in Israeli children: parents' answers to an epidemiological questionnaire. Public Health Rev 1990-1991;18: 335-344.

10. Ebomoyi EW. Pediculosis capitis among urban school children in Ilorin, Nigeria. J Natl Med Assoc 1994;86:861-864.

11. Busvine J. Pediculosis: biology of the parasites. In: Orkin M, Maibach H, editors. Cutaneous infestations and insect bites. New York: Marcel Dekker Inc.; 1985. p. 163-174.

12. Payot F. Contribution a l'etude du *Phthirus pubis* (Linne, Leach). Bull Soc Vaud Natl 1920;53:127-161.

13. Takano-Lee M, Yoon KS, Edman JD, Mullens BA, Clark JM. *In vivo* and *in vitro* rearing of *Pediculus humanus capitis* (Anoplura: Pediculidae). J Med Entomol 2003;40:628-635.

14. Takano-Lee M, Edman JD, Mullens BA, Clark JM. Transmission potential of the human head louse, *Pediculus capitis* (Anoplura: Pediculidae). Int J Dermatol 2005;44:811-816.

15. Speare R, Cahill C, Thomas G. Head lice on pillows, and strategies to make a small risk even less. Int J Dermatol 2003;42:626-629.

16. Speare R, Buettner PG. Hard data needed on head lice transmission. Int J Dermatol 2000;39:877-878.

17. Speare R, Thomas G, Cahill C. Head lice are not found on floors in primary school classrooms. Aust NZ J Public Health 2002;26:208-211.

18. Andrews JR, Tonkin SL. Scabies and pediculosis in Tokelau Island children in New Zealand. J R Soc Health 1989;109:199-203.

19. Kwaku-Kpikpi JE. The incidence of the head louse (*Pediculus humanus capitis*) among pupils of two schools in Accra. Trans R Soc Trop Med Hyg 1982;76: 378-381.

20. Sinniah B, Chandra S, Ramphal L, Senan P. Pediculosis among rural school children in Kelang, Selangor, Malaysia and their susceptibility to malathion, carbaryl, perigen and kerosene. Journal of the Royal Society of Health 1984;104:114-115, 118.

21. Jinadu MK. Pediculus humanus capitis among primary school children in Ife-Ife, Nigeria. J R Soc Health 1985;105:25-27.

22. Chunge R. A study of head lice among primary school children in Kenya. Trans R Soc Trop Med Hyg 1986;80: 42-46.

23. Chunge R, Scott F, Underwood J, Zavarella K. A review of the epidemiology, public health importance, treatment and control of head lice. Can J Public Health 1991;82:196-200.

24. Chunge RN, Scott FE, Underwood JE, Zavarella KJ. A pilot study to investigate transmission of headlice. Can J Public Health 1991;82:207-208.

25. CDC. Head lice treatment. Atlanta, GA USA: Centres for Disease Control and Prevention; 2008 [updated 07/10/08; cited 2009 14 September]; Available from: http://www.cdc.gov/lice/head/treatment.html.

26. Maunder JW. The appreciation of lice. Proc R Inst G B 1983;55:1-31.

27. Burgess IF. Human lice and their management. Adv Parasitol 1995;36:271-342.

28. Speare R, Buettner PG. Head lice in pupils of a primary school in Australia and implications for control. Int J Dermatol 1999;38:285-290.

29. Canyon DV, Speare R, Muller R. Spatial and kinetic factors for the transfer of head lice (*Pediculus capitis*) between hairs. J Invest Dermatol 2002; 119:629-631.

30. Mumcuoglu K, Miller J, Gofin R, Adler B, Ben-Ishai F, Almog R, et al. Epidemiological studies on head lice infestation in Israel. I. Parasitological examination of children. Int J Dermatol 1990;29:502-506.

31. Speare R, Ahn S. Eradicating head lice in a nursing home. Aust Fam Physician 1999;28:915-917.

32. Counahan M, Andrews R, Büttner P, Byrnes G, Speare R. Head lice prevalence in primary schools in Victoria, Australia. J Paediatr Child Health 2004;40:616-619.

33. Heukelbach J, Winter B, Wilcke T, Muehlen M, Albrecht S, de Oliveira FA, et al. Selective mass treatment with ivermectin to control intestinal helminthiases and parasitic skin diseases in a severely affected population. Bull World Health Organ 2004;82:563-571.

34. Sinniah B, Sinniah D, Rajeswari B. Epidemiology and control of human head louse in Malaysia. Trop Geogr Med 1983;35:337-342.

35. Maunder J. An update on head lice. Health Visit 1993;66:317-318.

36. Maunder B. Attitude to head lice - a more powerful force than insecticides. J R Soc Health 1985;105:61-64.

37. Wickenden J. The life and habits of the head louse. Midwife Health Visit Community Nurse 1984;20:368.

3.2. Prevalence and incidence of head lice

3.2.1. Prevalence

Head lice are cosmopolitan insects, and infestations are prevalent throughout the world. Prevalence varies considerably among populations, gender, age groups and according to behavioural factors within a population. In general, head lice are more common at younger age and in females. It is commonly accepted that girls have a higher prevalence of infestation due to playing with each other more closely than age-matched boys. Independent of socio-cultural settings, prevalence of infestation may be high. During recent years, anecdotal evidence suggested that the prevalence has increased worldwide, mainly in resource-rich countries [1].

There is quite an extensive list of studies aiming at the description of prevalence of head lice from all continents. However, most studies are historical, and methods to detect infestations differ considerably between surveys, which makes comparison of results difficult [1, 2]. In addition, many studies were performed in schoolchildren or in high risk populations (such as refugees, urban slums, jails, orphanages), and only few studies were community-based. In general, reported prevalences in Europe are lower than from other parts of the World. Nevertheless, the available evidence shows clearly that head lice are prevalent in both developed market economies and resource-poor countries.

In fact, reported prevalences differ widely, from less than 2% in children from Korea, Germany and Poland to about 60% in Nepalese street children and Argentinian schoolchildren [1, 3-5]. A cross-sectional study from Belgium in more than 6,000 children detected a prevalence of 9% by wet combing [6]. Similar to other studies, infestation was significantly more common in girls [6-8]. In Braunschweig, Germany, the point prevalence as detected by health services during preschool screening (1890 children aged 5-6 years) was 0.7% [4]. As diagnosis was made by visual inspection, a rather insensitive diagnostic method (☞ Chapter 5.1.), true prevalence was expected to range between 2 and 3%. Six per cent of children had been infested in the previous 12 months [4]. Data from the UK have shown that in some communities in Europe prevalences may reach astonishingly high rates. For example, in Bristol primary schoolchildren, about 40% of girls aged 6-7 years were found infested [9]. A questionnaire-based study from the UK has shown that 37% of more than 20,000 schoolchildren were infested during the period of a year [10].

In a population-based study in Brazil, prevalence (detected by visual inspection) was 43% in an urban slum and 28% in a fishing community [7]. In girls living in the urban slum, prevalence was higher than 80%.

In areas in Africa where severe infectious diseases such as malaria are endemic, head lice are often not perceived as a health problem, but as a nuisance [11]. However, there are also areas in northern Africa, as well as in sub-Saharan Africa, where pediculosis is endemic [2]. Similarly to other parts of the world, prevalence studies from these areas are mainly based on school populations. For example, in two studies performed in the 1980s (Cameroon and Ghana), 32% of more than 2300 schoolchildren and 49% of 319 schoolchildren were infested, respectively [12, 13]. Similarly, children from Egypt were reported having high rates of infestation [1]. In a rural community in Nigeria, overall prevalence in the population was recently reported to be 29% [11]. On the other hand, in a school in South Africa, head lice were not detected in black school children, whereas prevalence in the white ethnic group was 16% [2].

3.2.2. Seasonal variation

Seasonal variation of the occurrence of head lice infestations does not follow a clear pattern when compared between countries, and is usually claimed to be lower during school holidays with outbreaks after children return to school [5, 14]. In Germany, the number of head lice consultations in a community Health Department was lower during school holidays, with an increase when school started [15]. The number of pediculicides sold in late summer/early autumn was found to double after summer holidays. The authors suggested that during summer months and summer holidays travel increases the likelihood that other children from different geographic areas come in contact, which would facilitate dissemination of the parasites [15]. In addition, people may simply not seek medical care during holidays. In soldiers of the Israeli Army, the number of head lice infestations increased clearly during summer months [16]. In Brazil, community-based prevalences ranged between 44% in March (rainy season) and 27% in September (dry season) [7]. The reasons for seasonal variations are still not clear and may include climatic, environmental, behavioural and cultural factors, besides the pattern of school holidays.

3.2.3. Incidence

Incidence of head lice infestations has rarely been assessed systematically. In Germany, the incidence in preschool children (5-6 years of age) was estimated to be around 600 cases per 10,000 children per year [4]. In a community-based study from an urban slum in Brazil, incidence was assessed in children and teenagers after rigorous specific head lice treatment of affected individuals [17]. The median infestation-free time was only 14 days (interquartile range: 11-25 days). After 30 days, already 79% of individuals were reinfested, with higher rates in females.

In conclusion, the prevalence of head lice is high and seems to rise across most parts of the world.

3.2.4. References

1. Falagas ME, Matthaiou DK, Rafailidis PI, Panos G, Pappas G. Worldwide prevalence of head lice. Emerg Infect Dis 2008;14:1493-1494.

2. Govere JM, Speare R, Durrheim DN. The prevalence of pediculosis in rural South African schoolchildren. S Afr J Sci 2003;99:21-23.

3. Buczek A, Markowska-Gosik D, Widomska D, Kawa IM. Pediculosis capitis among schoolchildren in urban and rural areas of eastern Poland. Eur J Epidemiol 2004; 19:491-495.

4. Jahnke C, Bauer E, Feldmeier H. [Pediculosis capita in childhood: epidemiological and socio-medical results from screening of school beginners]. Gesundheitswesen (Bundesverband der Ärzte des Öffentlichen Gesundheitsdienstes/Germany) 2008;70:667-673.

5. Richter J, Müller-Stöver I, Walter S, Mehlhorn H, Häussinger D. Kopfläuse - Umgang mit einer wieder auflebenden Parasitose. Dtsch Arztebl 2005;102: 2395-2398.

6. Willems S, Lapeere H, Haedens N, Pasteels I, Naeyaert JM, De Maeseneer J. The importance of socio-economic status and individual characteristics on the prevalence of head lice in schoolchildren. Eur J Dermatol 2005;15:387-392.

7. Heukelbach J, Wilcke T, Winter B, Feldmeier H. Epidemiology and morbidity of scabies and pediculosis capitis in resource-poor communities in Brazil. Br J Dermatol 2005;153:150-156.

8. Catala S, Junco L, Vaporaky R. *Pediculus capitis* infestation according to sex and social factors in Argentina. Rev Saude Publica 2005;39:438-443.

9. Downs AM, Stafford KA, Coles GC. Head lice: prevalence in schoolchildren and insecticide resistance. Parasitol Today 1999;15:1-4.

10. Harris J, Crawshaw JG, Millership S. Incidence and prevalence of head lice in a district health authority area. Communicable disease and public health / PHLS 2003;6: 246-249.

11. Ugbomoiko US, Speare R, Heukelbach J. Self-diagnosis of head lice infestation in rural Nigeria as a reliable rapid assessment tool for pediculosis. The Open Dermatology Journal 2008;2:95-97.

12. Awahmukalah DS, Dinga JS, Nchako NJ. Pediculosis among urban and rural school children in Kumba, Meme division, south-west Cameroon. Parassitologia 1988;30:249-256.

13. Kwaku-Kpikpi JE. The incidence of the head louse (*Pediculus humanus capitis*) among pupils of two schools in Accra. Trans R Soc Trop Med Hyg 1982;76: 378-381.

14. Weir E. School's back, and so is the lowly louse. CMAJ 2001;165:814.

15. Bauer E, Jahnke C, Feldmeier H. Seasonal fluctuations of head lice infestation in Germany. Parasitol Res. 2009;104:677-681.

16. Mimouni D, Ankol OE, Gdalevich M, Grotto I, Davidovitch N, Zangvil E. Seasonality trends of *Pediculosis capitis* and *Phthirus pubis* in a young adult population: follow-up of 20 years. J Eur Acad Dermatol Venereol. 2002;16:257-259.

17. Pilger D, Heukelbach J, Khakban A, Oliveira FA, Fengler G, Feldmeier H. Impact of household-wide treatment for the control of head lice infestations in an impoverished community: randomized observer-blinded comparative trial. Bull World Health Organ 2010;88: 90-96.

Clinical Aspects

4. Clinical Aspects

4.1. Symptoms

Many patients remain asymptomatic. Pruritus, an immune-mediated reaction to components of lice saliva, is the most common symptom of head lice infestations. The degree of itching seems to increase with the duration of infestation and the number of lice present on the scalp, but may depend also on the socio-cultural setting. In two endemic communities in Brazil, itching was the predominant symptom, but intensity was generally perceived as low [1]. In Venezuela, 18% of infested schoolchildren reported itching [2]. In France, itching was reported in 14% of schoolchildren with head lice [3], whereas in Israel, about 30% of infested children complained about itching—but 23% did not show any symptoms or signs [4].

Similar to other skin diseases, the intensity of itching is significantly higher during the first three hours of sleep. As a consequence children with pediculosis capitis often complain about sleep disturbances [5]. We assume that the threshold of the itch sensation is downregulated at night, as observed in other skin diseases [6]. Persistent disturbance of sleep may lead to concentration problems, tiredness and poor performance in school [7].

4.2. Signs

Clinical findings in head lice infestation can be differentiated into primary and secondary signs.

Primary signs are reddish, intensively itching papules of 2-3 mm diameter, most frequently in the retro-auricular region of the scalp. They are often surrounded by an erythema. Immediately after a bite wheals may occur, with the subsequent development of papules and itching.

In the case of primary infestation, these signs develop with a delay of 4-6 weeks. In the case of re-infestation, signs appear within 24-48 hours—an indicator for an immune-mediated reaction against components of lice saliva. Presumably, this is a delayed-type hypersensitivity reaction similar to the one observed in scabies and bed bug infestations [6, 8].

Secondary signs are the result of extensive scratching of the scalp. Repeated scratching leads to excoriations in the epidermis (☞ Figure 4.1). If the patient is not treated and continues scratching, ulcers may develop [9]. Excoriations reduce the natural barrier function of the epidermis and are an entry port for pathogenic microorganisms, typically *Staphylococcus aureus* and streptococci, leading to impetiginisation of the scalp (☞ Figure 4.2). Head lice may carry passively these bacteria from infected to healthy areas of the scalp [5]. Persistent infection with group A streptococci may pose the patient at risk for post-streptococcal glomerulonephritis.

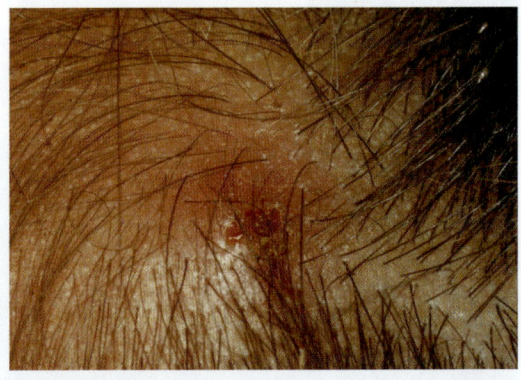

Figure 4.1: Excoriation of the scalp surrounded by an erythema.

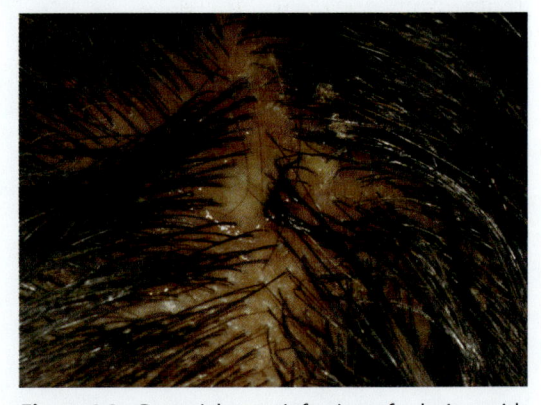

Figure 4.2: Bacterial superinfection of a lesion with *Staphylococcus aureus* in a child infested with head lice.

In two resource-poor communities in Brazil, bacterial superinfection was observed in about 3% of infested individuals [1]. In a study in France, only

1.2% of children with pediculosis capitis showed signs of superinfection [3]. In German pre-school children, the frequency of superinfection was even less common [10].

Persistent superinfection leads to the development of regional lymphadenopathy. In two populations with repeated head lice infestations and a restricted access to health care, cervical lymphadenopathy was observed in 12% and 15% of infested individuals [1]. In an endemic setting in Venezuela with intense transmission, lymphadenopathy occurred in 7.3% of infested children, compared to 5.5% in noninfested individuals [2]. In Israel, the frequency of lymphadenopathy in infested children (at any topographic site) was 60% (and 54% in non-infested individuals) [4]. In a historical report from Germany, Brusis and Unshelm (1977) observed cervical lymphadenopathy in 11% of patients with head lice infestations [11].

Chronic infestations and persistent scratching may lead to eczema of the scalp ("lice eczema"), most commonly located in the neck [4, 12]. Excoriation and eczematisation may considerably increase the absorption of topically applied pediculicides. This is of particular importance when neurotoxic compounds are applied topically [13].

Salamon & Lazovic-Tepavac (1970) reported focal alopecia in two heavily infested children which developed after treatment [14]. These patients showed hypochromic anaemia, leukocytosis and relative lymphocytosis. Meinking (1996) observed similar alterations in heavily infested individuals in the USA [5]. In fact, persistent heavy infestation with hundreds of head lice has been considered to cause anaemia in single cases [15, 16].

Mumcuoglu et al. (1991) documented conjunctivitis in 54.1% of infested children, but failed to provide a pathophysiological basis for this observation and did not report the frequency of this sign in non-infested children [4]. Cazorla et al. (2007) did not observe any difference in the occurrence of conjunctivitis between infested and non-infested schoolchildren [2].

In rare cases, chronic impetiginisation of the scalp associated with massive exsudation, resulting in hair shafts intricately glued to each other (similar to the Polish plait observed in the 19th century), can be seen in homeless children or neglected children refugees in low income countries.

4.3. References

1. Heukelbach J, Wilcke T, Winter B, Feldmeier H. Epidemiology and morbidity of scabies and pediculosis capitis in resource-poor communities in Brazil. Br J Dermatol 2005;153:150-156.

2. Cazorla D, Ruiz A, Acosta M. [Clinical and epidemiological study of pediculosis capitis in schoolchildren from Coro, Venezuela]. Invest Clin 2007;48: 445-457.

3. Courtiade C, Labreze C, Fontan I, Taieb A, Maleville J. [Pediculosis capitis: a questionnaire survey in 4 schools of the Bordeaux Academy 1990-1991]. Ann Dermatol Venereol 1993;120:363-368.

4. Mumcuoglu KY, Klaus S, Kafka D, Teiler M, Miller J. Clinical observations related to head lice infestation. J Am Acad Dermatol 1991;25:248-251.

5. Meinking TL, Taplin D. Infestations: pediculosis. Curr Probl Dermatol 1996;24:157-163.

6. Hon KL, Lam MC, Leung TF, Chik KW, Leung AK. A malignant itch. J Nat Med Assoc 2006;98:1992-1994.

7. Heukelbach J, Feldmeier H. Ectoparasites—the underestimated realm. Lancet 2004;363:889-891.

8. Leverkus M, Jochim RC, Schad S, Brocker EB, Andersen JF, Valenzuela JG, et al. Bullous allergic hypersensitivity to bed bug bites mediated by IgE against salivary nitrophorin. J Invest Dermatol 2006;126:91-96.

9. Feldmeier H. Pediculosis capitis - Die wichtigste Parasitose des Kindesalters. Kinder- und Jugendmedizin 2006;4:249-259.

10. Jahnke C, Bauer E, Feldmeier H. Pediculosis capita in childhood: epidemiological and socio-medical results from screening of school beginners. Gesundheitswesen 2008;70:667-673.

11. Brusis T, Unshelm W. Klinik und Therapie der Pedikulosen. Dtsch Arztebl 1977;5:293-298.

12. Hamm H. Mites, lice and fleas. Ectoparasitoses in infancy and childhood. Hautarzt 2005;56:915-924.

13. Tomalik-Scharte D, Lazar A, Meins J, Bastian B, Ihrig M, Wachall B, et al. Dermal absorption of permethrin following topical administration. Europ J Clin Pharmacol 2005;61:399-404.

14. Salamon T, Lazovic-Tepavac O. Circumscribing alopecia caused by head lice. Dermatol Monatsschr 1970; 156:676-682.

15. Speare R, Canyon DV, Melrose W. Quantification of blood intake of the head louse: *Pediculus humanus capitis*. Int J Dermatol 2006;45:543-546.

16. Linardi PM, Neves DP, de Melo AL, Genaro O, Linardi PM. Anoplura. Parasitologia humana. São Paulo, Rio de Janeiro, Belo Horizonte: Editora Atheneu; 2002. p. 368-372.

Diagnosis and Rapid Assessment

5. Diagnosis and Rapid Assessment

5.1. Diagnosis of head lice infestations

A correct diagnosis is the prerequisite for appropriate treatment. People with active pediculosis have live lice on the scalp or live embryos in eggs attached to hair shafts. People with inactive pediculosis have no live lice, but dead eggs or egg shells (nits) are found on hair shafts [1].

An active head lice infestation bears risk of transmission and requires treatment. In contrast, inactive pediculosis is only evidence of past infection. There is no transmission risk, but it often is a cosmetic, social, mental and economic problem [1]. In this situation, removal of egg shells becomes the major goal.

However, in clinical praxis, it is difficult to conclude whether a patient has an active infestation or shows only residues from pediculosis experienced in the past. This is due to the fact that infestation intensity is low in many cases (≤10 trophic stages). In addition, laymen and doctors usually are unable to differentiate viable ova, dead ova or nits. Finally, diagnostic techniques need certain skills and are time-consuming.

5.1.1. Diagnosis of active infestation

Diagnosis of an active infestation is made when a living louse is found. Usually, this diagnosis is made by visual inspection: Direct observation of adult parasites or nymphs on the scalp. After parting the hair (e.g. with an applicator stick), the scalp is examined systematically, preferably with an illuminated magnifying glass. Predilection sites are the areas behind the ears and the neck. This method requires only minimal resources and is easy to perform.

However, visual inspection is an insensitive method, even when the whole scalp is inspected [2-4]. In one study, in only 6% of children head lice were found on the scalp by visual inspection, as compared to 25% after detection combing, resulting in a sensitivity of visual inspection of 22% [5]. More recent data from Turkey and Germany revealed similar low sensitivities of 31% and 29%, as compared to wet combing [3, 4]. These studies showed that visual inspection underestimates the prevalence of active pediculosis by a factor 3-4. Consequently, in developed market economies visual inspection cannot be recommended as a diagnostic means to diagnose active infestation.

The situation is different in resource-poor settings in the developing world, where infestation intensity is high and mothers are daily confronted with head lice infestations of their offspring. For instance, mothers living in a slum in Brazil, who screened the heads of their children regularly, performed visual inspection with a sensitivity of 43% [6]. In a population-based study in an endemic community the sensitivity of visual inspection performed by mothers of affected children was 35%, with 100% specificity [7].

A very simple approach to diagnose active head lice infestation is asking individuals about their infestation status. This approach has been used in resource-poor areas where people commonly have head lice, but no adequate access to health care. Caretakers in poor communities in Brazil and Nigeria, after being asked about the presence of head lice on the head of their children, were aware of the infestation status with a sensitivity of 74-81% for active infestation [7, 8]. In the case of severe infestation, the sensitivity of self-diagnosis was as high as 92% in the Nigerian study.

The most reliable method to diagnose active head lice infestation is by detection combing. Detection combing can be performed on dry or wet hair. Combs must have parallel-sided teeth and a distance of ≤0.3 mm between teeth, so that small first instar nymphs are caught between the teeth (☞ Chapter 6.1. for details).

Wet combing can be considered as the gold standard. A conditioner is applied onto the hair first. Lice enter into stasis, do not crawl away and therefore stick to the comb and are easily detected in the conditioner liquid. After each strike, the conditioner is wiped on sanitary paper to detect objects stuck between the teeth of the comb (☞ Figures 5.1a+b). Combing has to be done systematically from one side of the head to the other. The sensitivity of systematic wet combing in children with a low infestation intensity is in the order of 90%, and in patients with more than 10 trophic stages it is

5.1. Diagnosis of head lice infestations

considered to be almost 100% [4]. However, since this method needs skilled personnel and is more resource-intensive than dry combing, its use in screening programs is limited [9].

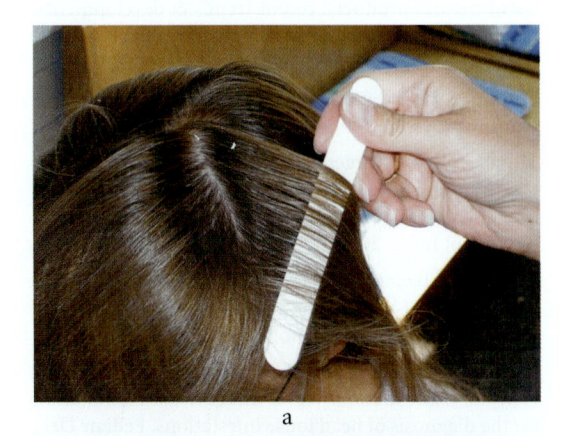

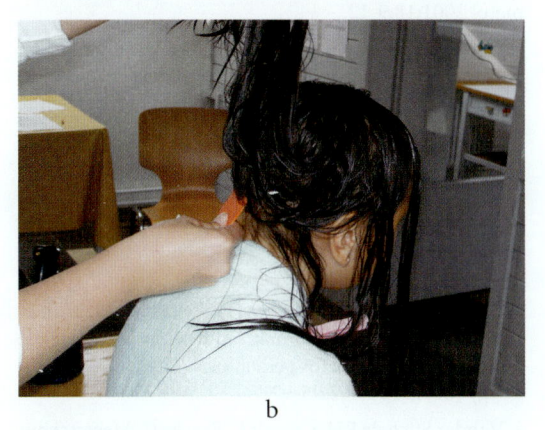

Figure 5.1a+b: Wet combing using an applicator stick and a fine toothed comb. Images: H. Feldmeier, Germany.

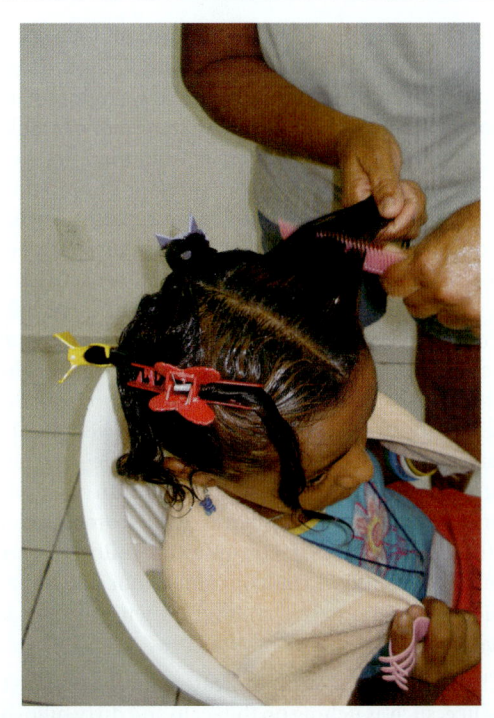

Figure 5.2: If hair is long, hair clips may also be used to facilitate wet combing. Image: J. Heukelbach, Brazil.

As head lice can be identified with the naked eye and cannot be confounded with artefacts, the specificity of visual inspection and of detection combing should be very high. However, diagnosis of head lice infestations is often done by people who are not used with size and shape of head lice and consequently misinterpret what they see. In the USA, only 59% of 614 samples sent to a reference centre for diagnosis of head lice infestation, contained trophic forms or eggs [10]. Surprisingly, only 17% of samples forwarded by physicians contained louse-derived material, as compared to 70% from nurses and 86% from teachers [10]. Debris such as dandruff, and other epidermal material was found in 35% of all samples, other arthropods (book lice, beetles mites, bed bugs etc.) in 5%, and knotted hair in one sample. In addition, only 53% of the specimens thought to contain a trophic stage or a viable egg actually showed the corresponding life stages of the parasite. The remaining samples contained mostly nits, indicating an infestation in the past. Neurotoxic pediculicides were applied by 62% to individuals with specimens without lice material, indicating unnecessary treatment in a considerable number of cases [10].

It has been suggested to use the distance of eggs to the scalp as a proxy of their viability. This is based on the assumption that within 10 days nymphs are hatched from viable eggs and that the hair of a child grows approximately 10 mm per month. Eggs seen more than 10 mm away from the scalp should thus not contain viable embryos. In a reverse conclusion, eggs cemented to a hair shaft in proximity to the scalp were considered to indicate an active infestation. However, only a small percentage of children with eggs close to the scalp actually have an active infestation. In one study, only 18% of the children with eggs cemented within 6 mm from the scalp—but without lice—actually showed lice 14 days later [11]. These data show that the presence of eggs near to the scalp cannot be used to conclude on active head lice infestation. Data from another study suggested that non-infested children were more frequently excluded from school due to pediculosis than infested children, when diagnosis is based on the presence of nits [10].

There are other indirect indicators for the presence of lice, such as itching on the scalp and dirty pillows in the morning, but none of them is accurate enough to base therapy on. Itching of the scalp may have other causes than head lice such as eczema or mosquito bites. The presence of infestation in other family members, though, with concurrent presence of one or more of these signs is sufficient to initiate specific treatment.

5.1.2. Diagnosis of historical infestation

The diagnosis of historical head lice infestation is made by the detection of egg shells or dead eggs. This information is useful to track transmission during outbreaks in a kindergarten or a school, or to determine the period prevalence of head lice infestation in a population group.

With regard to the detection of eggs, visual inspection is superior as compared with wet combing (sensitivity 86% versus 68%). However, if only a few eggs are present, these are often overlooked by visual inspection, but confirmed by wet combing, and the accuracy of both methods is rather similar (96% versus 92%) [4]. Since visual inspection is rapidly done, requires no additional resources other than a reusable applicator stick, this technique is the method of choice if the frequency of historical pediculosis capitis is to be determined.

5.1.3. References

1. Heukelbach J, Speare R, Canyon D. Natural products and their application to the control of head lice: an evidence-based review. In: Brahmachari G, editor. Chemistry of natural products: recent trends & developments. First ed. Kerala, India: Research Signpost; 2006. p. 277-302.

2. Burgess IF. Human lice and their management. Adv Parasitol 1995;36:271-342.

3. Balcioglu C, Burgess IF, Limoncu ME, Sahin MT, Ozbel Y, Bilac C, et al. Plastic detection comb better than visual screening for diagnosis of head louse infestation. Epidemiol Infect 2008:1-7.

4. Jahnke C, Bauer E, Hengge UR, Feldmeier H. Accuracy of diagnosis of pediculosis capitis: visual inspection vs wet combing. Arch Dermatol 2009;145:309-313.

5. Mumcuoglu KY, Friger M, Ioffe-Uspensky I, Ben Ishai F, Miller J. Louse comb versus direct visual examination for the diagnosis of head louse infestations. Pediatr Dermatol 2001;18:9-12.

6. Heukelbach J, Kuenzer M, Counahan M, Feldmeier H, Speare R. Correct diagnosis of current head lice infestation made by affected individuals from a hyperendemic area. Int J Dermatol 2006;45:1437-1438.

7. Pilger D, Khakban A, Heukelbach J, Feldmeier H. Self-diagnosis of active head lice infestation by individuals from an impoverished community: high sensitivity and specificity. Rev Inst Med Trop Sao Paulo 2008;50:121-122.

8. Ugbomoiko US, Speare R, Heukelbach J. Self-diagnosis of head lice infestation in rural Nigeria as a reliable rapid assessment tool for pediculosis. The Open Dermatology Journal 2008;2:95-97.

9. Vander Stichele RH, Gyssels L, Bracke C, Meersschaut F, Blokland I, Wittouck E, et al. Wet combing for head lice: feasibility in mass screening, treatment preference and outcome. J Royal Soc Med 2002;95:348-352.

10. Pollack RJ, Kiszewski AE, Spielman A. Overdiagnosis and consequent mismanagement of head louse infestations in North America. Pediatr Infect Dis J 2000;19:689-693.

11. Williams LK, Reichert A, MacKenzie WR, Hightower AW, Blake PA. Lice, nits, and school policy. Pediatrics 2001;107:1011-1015.

5.2. Rapid assessment of head lice infestations

When financial and human resources are limited, policy makers and health care providers need cost-effective and simple indicators for health problems. The so-called rapid assessment method is a way to investigate situations in which some issues are not yet well defined and where sufficient time or resources for long-term assessments are not given. In case of infectious and parasitic diseases, these simple indicators (such as asking a patient if he/she considers being infected, or simple clinical assessments) are commonly used to plan and monitor mass interventions. Additionally, rapid assessment also helps to detect parasitised individuals, and to plan individual treatment. Rapid assessment methods have been developed for a variety of diseases and health conditions, and thus have a great value in resource-poor as well as in high income settings [1-4]. These methods may also be helpful to plan and monitor interventions.

The most appropriate way to detect infestation in an individual would be asking that person about his/her infestation status. In endemic communities people usually know head lice and are aware of their infestation and accuracy of this approach is expected to be high. However, the value of self-diagnosis of pediculosis varies greatly with geographic locations and populations [5-8].

Two studies from Brazil have shown that people in urban endemic communities diagnosed their own head lice infestations with high positive predictive values of 89% and 98%, respectively [7, 8]. In contrast, sensitivity of visual inspection in these populations was only 35% and 43%.

One study from Nigeria assessed self-diagnosis of individuals. In a rural community, accuracy of self-diagnosing head lice infestations was high. Sensitivity was 74%, specificity 99% and the positive predictive value 97%. In individuals with heavy infestation, sensitivity was even increased to 92% [9].

On the other hand, in Australia sensitivity of parental diagnosis of head lice in children was very low (16%), with a positive predictive value of 67% [6]. In Mexico schoolchildren self-diagnosing pediculosis had also a low sensitivity, even though they were asked about the presence of nits, and not of active infestations [5].

As a consequence, in Brazil and Nigeria, treatment of head lice infestations could be based on self-diagnosis, and there is no need for resource-intensive and unnecessary diagnosis by health professionals [7-9]. In Australia, parental reporting is not a reliable indicator of pediculosis [6]. This would also apply to the diagnostic accuracy of Mexican schoolchildren [5].

5.2.1. References

1. Anker M. Epidemiological and statistical methods for rapid health assessment: introduction. World Health Stat Q 1991;44:94-97.

2. Vlassoff C, Tanner M. The relevance of rapid assessment to health research and interventions. Health Policy Plan 1992;7:1-9.

3. Macintyre K. Rapid assessment and sample surveys: trade-offs in precision and cost. Health Policy Plan 1999;4:363-373.

4. Macintyre K, Bilsborrow RE, Olmedo C, Carrasco R. Rapid surveys for program evaluation: Design and implementation of an experiment in Ecuador. Rev Panam Salud Publica 1999;6:192-201.

5. Paredes SS, Estrada R, Alarcon H, Chavez G, Romero M, Hay R. Can school teachers improve the management and prevention of skin disease? A pilot study based on head louse infestations in Guerrero, Mexico. Int J Dermatol 1997;36:826-830.

6. Counahan ML, Andrews RM, Speare R. Reliability of parental reports of head lice in their children. Med J Aust 2005;82:137-138.

7. Heukelbach J, Kuenzer M, Counahan M, Feldmeier H, Speare R. Correct diagnosis of current head lice infestation made by affected individuals from a hyperendemic area. Int J Dermatol 2006;45:1437-1438.

8. Pilger D, Khakban A, Heukelbach J, Feldmeier H. Self-diagnosis of active head lice infestation by individuals from an impoverished community: high sensitivity and specificity. Rev Inst Med Trop Sao Paulo 2008;50:121-122.

9. Ugbomoiko US, Speare R, Heukelbach J. Self-diagnosis of head lice infestation in rural Nigeria as a reliable rapid assessment tool for pediculosis. The Open Dermatology Journal 2008;2:95-97.

Treatment Options and Resistance

6. Treatment Options and Resistance

6.1. Mechanical removal of lice and eggs

6.1.1. Lice and nit removal combs

The removal of head lice and lice eggs with a comb is one of the oldest known methods to control the infestation. Lice combs have been known for more than 3,500 years [1], and their design is actually very similar to some of those used today. Previously, the combs were made of natural materials like wood or horn (☞ Figure 6.1). Nowadays, a lice comb is typically designed in different types of plastic, metal or a combination of both (☞ Figure 6.2).

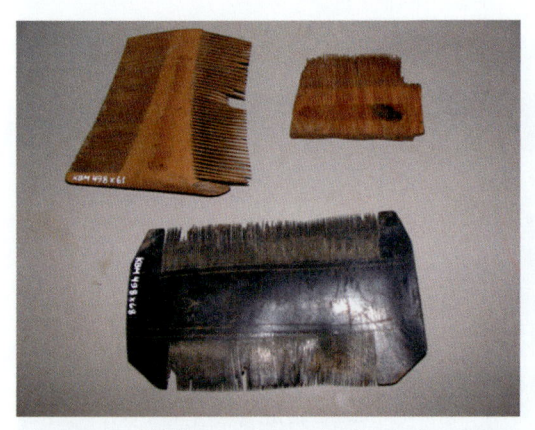

Figure 6.1: Old lice combs made of wood and horn (Image: K.S. Larsen, Denmark).

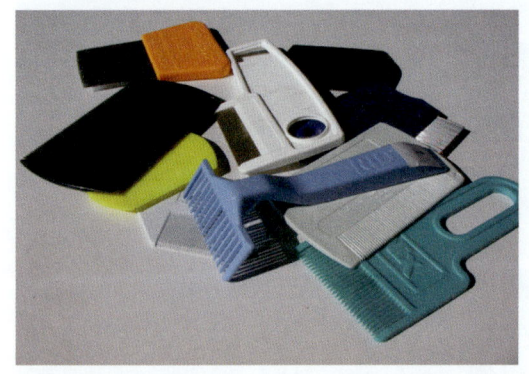

Figure 6.2: Modern lice combs (Image: K.S. Larsen, Denmark).

Especially after the occurrence of widespread resistance to many of the commonly used pediculicides it seemed that mechanical removal of lice by combing received a revival. Another major reason for the comb's success is based on the fact that an effective therapy requires a reliable diagnosis. The lice comb is, besides being a therapeutic tool, a vital instrument for detecting lice and thus an important diagnostic tool at the same time.

Most parents and professionals are familiar with lice combs, but very few people realise that the lice comb is a specialised tool that needs to meet specific requirements in order to detect and remove lice effectively. Unfortunately, no quality standards have been set for this type of combs, and only a limited number has actually been tested in adequately designed studies regarding their ability to remove lice or eggs. Nevertheless, there are some general recommendations to be considered before choosing a comb.

Normally, the effectiveness of fine-toothed combs depends on both the design and material. If the comb is made of plastic, a material of good quality should be used, for example acrylonitrile butadiene styrene (ABS) which is a resistant thermoplastic material and makes the teeth strong and flexible at the same time. Soft teeth will bend too easily and allow the lice to escape during the combing process, whereas combs with metal pins do not have this problem. The comb or rather its teeth can be tested by gently pushing the thumb along the row of teeth to check the quality.

The colour of the comb is of certain importance as well. When using a plastic comb in dry hair, a light-coloured comb is generally preferred, making it fairly easy to recognise the darker lice. When using a hair conditioner (wet-combing) in order to facilitate the combing process, the colour of the comb is of less importance as the remains of the hair conditioner on the comb is normally wiped off with a piece of soft paper to check for lice.

Combs intended for removing lice eggs need to have a small distance between the teeth. On average, a louse egg is 0.33 mm wide, but relatively flexible. Consequently, eggs and empty eggs (nits) will not be removed if the gap between the teeth is too wide and/or the design of the teeth is not optimal (☞ Figure 6.3). A comb used for the detection and removal of nymphs and adult lice should have a distance between the teeth of 0.2-0.3 mm, preferably close to 0.2 mm to remove even small first stage nymphs.

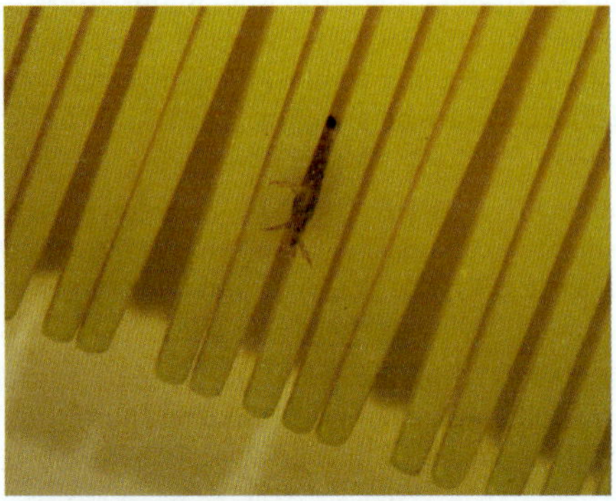

Figure 6.3: Adult louse caught between the teeth of a comb (Image: K.S. Larsen, Denmark).

Only few studies have been performed to compare the efficacy of different types of combs in their ability to remove lice and/or their eggs. In Table 6.1 the influence that material and design might have on combing results is demonstrated. Different types of combs (tested *in vitro*) are shown and their very different abilities to remove the empty lice eggs [2]. The data clearly demonstrate that the effectiveness of a specific comb to remove eggs depends not only on the distance between the teeth but also on the shape, material and fabric of the teeth.

Comb	Tooth gap (µm)	± [SD]	Empty eggs removed
Nix	61	[10]	100%
Innomed	146	[10]	85%
LiceMeister	99	[23]	55%
Napp	241	[15]	50%
Step 2	160	[8]	50%
Medicis	160	[8]	45%
Rid	152	[40]	30%
Dust comb	151	[12]	30%
Gicli	170	[48]	20%
Clear	211	[16]	20%
Bugbuster	265	[80]	20%
Pin comb	209	[12]	5%

Table 6.1: The ability of different combs to remove empty lice eggs (data taken from [2]).

A limited number of clinical studies support these data. In one clinical study, three types of plastic combs were compared. Following the use of a pediculicide, the participants were combed with different combs on the right and left halves of the head. No differences were observed in the ability of the three combs to remove head lice; however, one comb was significantly better in removing eggs [3]. In another study, the efficacy of a metal pin comb and a plastic comb was compared, regarding their ability to remove both lice and eggs. The efficacy of the combs was again assessed by using a different comb on the right and left halves of the head. There was no significant difference in their ability to remove lice, but the metal pin comb (LiceMeister) removed more eggs than the plastic comb (Lady Jane comb) [4]. In both studies lice and eggs were removed after treatment with pediculicides.

In general, removal of eggs is commonly believed to be an important part of the treatment strategy for head lice, due to the fact that pediculicides may not kill all eggs. In fact, many producers of pediculicides include a comb in the package. The removal of eggs or regular wet combing alone have been promoted as an adequate therapy [6, 7]. One study evaluated the efficacy of 1% permethrin with and without the adjunctive daily removal of lice and eggs [6]. There was no benefit obtained from adjunctive combing. In this study, the assessment at day 8 found that nearly 46% of those who received the pediculicide treatment alone were free of lice compared to 33% of those using adjunctive combing. At day 15, the combing group had a higher treatment failure compared to the group treated with permethrin only (72.7% versus 78.3%), although the difference was not statistically significant. A couple of other studies compared the efficacy of pediculicide treatment with regular combing [7-9]. The method of combing tested is called "bug busting" (BB) which is based on a methodical removal of lice, but not their eggs. It consists of wet combing with a hair conditioner, carried out on day 1, 5, 9 and 13. In one study [8], two applications seven days apart of 0.5% malathion performed better than BB (78% versus 38% cure). In return, however, another study showed that only 13% were cured, when using two applications of 0.2% phenothrin, as compared to 53% in the BB group [9]. Additionally, one study compared a single treatment of 0.5% malathion or 1%

permethrin with the BB therapy. The cure rate for the pediculicides showed 13% in total versus 57% for the BB [7].

Apart from the "classical" combs mentioned above, other types of combs are available on the market. One type of comb is especially made to be mounted on a vacuum cleaner (The Licesnatcher), while others are electronic lice combs. The latter type is battery-powered and claims to "zap" the louse on the teeth of the comb. However, no efficacy trials have been published to support the use of any of these combs.

Although removal of lice using the "bug busting" method and the specific combs performed better than the pediculicidal treatments in two of the above mentioned studies, it demonstrates that the BB method has to be regarded as insufficient in the control of head lice. Combing as a method for treatment of a head louse infestation has been and may still be a cheap and proper alternative to the traditionally used pediculicides, especially in areas where resistance, as in the above mentioned studies, is present and thus demonstrating a lower efficacy compared to the combing. However, for combing to perform at the same level as the modern physically acting pediculicides (containing e.g. fatty acid esters and/or silicones) with cure rates between 77% and as high as 97% [10-14] there is a need for future studies to evaluate the efficacy of combing and its variations, e.g. wet combing versus dry combing, increased frequency and the use of new types of lice combs.

6.1.2. References

1. Mumcuoglu KY, Zias J. Head Lice, *Pediculus humanus capitis* (Anoplura: Pediculidae), from hair Combs Excavated in Israel and Dated from First Century B.C. to Eighth century A.D. J Med Entomol 1988;25:545-547.

2. Larsen KS, Burgess I. Combs for removing lice and nits. In: Barker S, Ellender C, editors. Proceedings of the 2nd International Congress on Phthiraptera; 2002 July 8-12; Brisbane, Australia. Brisbane; 2002. p. 64.

3. de Souza Bueno V, de Oliveira Garcia L, de Oliveira NJ, da Silva Ribeiro, DC. Comparative study on the efficiency of three different fine-tooth combs to remove lice and nits. Rev Bras Med 2001;58.

4. Speare R, Canyon DV, Cahill C, Thomas G. Comparative efficacy of two nit combs in removing head lice (*Pediculus humanus* var. *capitis*) and their eggs. Int J Dermatol 2007;46:1275-1278.

5. Crossan, L. 2002. Experince based treatment of head lice. BMJ 324:1220.

6. Meinking TL, Clineschmidt CM, Chen C, Kolber MA, Tiping RW, Furtek CI et al. An observer-blinded study of 1% permathrin crème rinse with and without adjunctive combing in patients with head lice. J Pediatr 2002;141:665-670.

7. Hill N, Moor G, Cameron MN, Butlin A, Preston S, Williason MS et al. Single blind, randomised, comparative study of the Bug Buster kit and over the counter pediculicide treatments against head lice in the United Kingdom. BMJ 2005;331:384-387.

8. Roberts RJ, Casey D, Morgan DA, Petrovic M. Comparison of wet combing with malathion for treatment of head lice in the UK: a pragmatic randomized controlled trial. Lancet 2000;356:540-544.

9. Plastow L, Luthra M, Powell R, Wright J, Russell D, Marshall MN. Head lice infestation: bug busting vs. traditional treatment. J Clin Nurs 2001;10:775-783.

10. Burgess IF, Lee PN, Matlock G. Randomised, controlled, assessor blind trial comparing 4% dimeticone lotion with 0.5% malathion liquid for head louse infestation. PLoS ONE 2007;2:e1127.

11. Kaul N, Palma KG, Silgay SS, Goodman JJ, Toole J. North American efficacy and safety of a novel pediculicide rinse, isopropyl myristate 50% (Resultz). J Cutan Med Surg 2007;11:161-167.

12. Burgess IF, Lee PN, Brown CM. Randomised, controlled, parallel group clinical trials to evaluate the efficacy of isopropyl myristate/cyclomethicone solution against head lice. Pharm J 2008;280:371-375.

13. Heukelbach J, Pilger D, Oliveira FA, et al. A highly efficacious pediculicide based on dimeticone: Randomised observer blinded comparative trial. BMC Infect Dis 2008; 8:115-124.

14. Burgess IF. Current treatments for pediculosis capitis. Curr Opin Infect Dis 2009;22:131-136

6.2. Treatments using pediculicides with neurotoxic mode of action

The most studied pediculicides are topical insecticides, including the more commonly used pyrethroids and organophosphates. These formulated insecticides are available for purchase in community pharmacies, with pyrethroids being the most widely used due to shorter contact time and less odour. Chemical insecticides are often still recommended as first-line treatment by national institutions. Nevertheless, new therapeutic strategies are evolving with the emergence of insecticide resistance and development of alternatives to classical pediculicidal agents (☞ Chapters 6.4. and 6.5.). As pediculicidal agents are sold over the counter (OTC), including the chemicals, there are no safeguards to prevent indiscriminate use of head-lice products. Efficacy depends on the insecticide itself and its formulation which may vary slightly by country. For example, the formulation of malathion in the United States and Europe contains terpenes that are suggested to have pediculicidal properties by itself [1]. An insecticide should theoretically have 100% killing activity against both lice and nits/eggs but some authors consider that available topical insecticides are poorly ovicidal [2]. Table 6.2 presents the most common pediculicides with neurotoxic mode of action.

6.2.1. Natural pyrethrins and semi-synthetic pyrethroids

Pyrethroids act primarily on the head lice nervous system ("knockdown" effect) where the target site is the voltage sensitive sodium channel. Permethrin can kill lice during the application and also has a long-lasting residual effect, which may be useful in killing nymphs emerging from eggs that were not killed. Paradoxically, these residual levels of permethrin may promote the emergence of resistance [3].

Natural pyrethrins or synthetic pyrethroids may be combined with an insecticide synergist (e.g. piperonyl butoxide). The duration of application depends on the molecule and its formulation (e.g. 10 minutes for permethrin or d-phenothrin). These products can be a fire hazard and burns have been reported, but they are cosmetically acceptable, and most adverse reactions are local and mild.

6.2.2. Organophosphates (malathion)

Malathion is an organophosphorous insecticide that irreversibly inhibits acetylcholinesterase, causing death by nerve hyper-excitability and exhaustion. It is relatively fast acting and the most effective ovicide among pediculicides [4].

Malathion is considered a safe treatment when the product is very pure and applied in accordance with the manufacturer's instructions. Although malathion is available since 1999 on the US market, it has been previously withdrawn twice because of its commercial failure (probably due to its odor, flammability, and long application time). Noteably, studies have shown that a 20-minute malathion treatment, instead of the approved 8- to 12-hour application, was effective [5, 6]. Malathion should not be used for children under 6 months.

6.2.3. Other insecticides

Lindane and DDT are neurotoxic for head lice, but an increasing number of countries have banned the medical use of lindane. Lindane is an organochlorine and, similar to DDT, can accumulate in

Group	Substance	Formulation	General comment	Efficacy	Main adverse events
Natural pyrethrins	Pyrethrin	± associated with a synergist like piperonyl butoxide	biodegradable	Very active fast knockdown	Low mammalian toxicity Skin irritation
Semi-synthetic pyrethrins (i.e. pyrethroids)	Permethrin, allethrin, deltamethrin, bioresmethrin, phenothrin,....	± associated with a synergist like piperonyl butoxide	Pyrethroids act on the head lice nervous system where the target site is the voltage sensitive sodium channel	More active than natural pyrethrins	Low mammalian toxicity Skin irritation May cause asthma attack
Organo-phosphates	Malathion	aqueous or alcoholic base	Irreversibly inhibits acetylcholinesterase causing death by nerve hyperexcitability	Fast acting, most effective ovicide	Skin irritation May cause asthma attack
Carbamates	Carbaryl	Carbaryl 1% in an aqueous basis	Restricted to physicians's prescription in the United Kingdom	Effective against adult stages	Carcinogenic effects to rodents

Table 6.2: Chemical treatments: formulations, general comments, efficacy and adverse events.

mammalian tissues. It also finds application as an insecticide in forestry and on fruit and vegetable crops for seed treatment. The European Union prohibited the use of lindane as an insecticide by the end of 2007. The chief advantage of lindane is its low cost but it is not used anymore in many countries because of concerns regarding neurotoxicity, resistance and slow killing time. Use of lindane is discouraged unless other treatments have failed or are intolerable.

Carbaryl's carcinogenicity has been demonstrated in rodents and is available on prescription only in the United Kingdom.

Topical crotamiton has been used in the past but there are limited data to support its efficacy.

6.2.4. Formulations and application

Lotions that deliver a high concentration of insecticides are preferable, but caution is required to avoid any contact with mucous membranes. Creams, foams, and gels are also available.

Insecticides should be applied to dry hair several times, as indicated by the manufacturer, in sufficient quantity. Application time depends on the formulation. Since neurotoxic insecticides are not 100% ovicidal, it is recommended to reapply pediculicidal treatment 7 to 11 days after the first application, thus killing newly hatched nymphs before they reach maturity and lay eggs.

Insecticide resistance is established in many countries, but treatment failure is often explained by poor treatment compliance or re-infestation. In fact, improper use of chemical pediculicide, like inadequate, incomplete or inappropriate applications, should be considered in case of treatment failure. The use of shampoos is not recommended, as they are diluted with water with a consequently lower concentration. Since in addition contact time of shampoos is short, they are less effective and may facilitate the emergence of resistance.

6.2.5. Adverse events and safety concerns

■ **General considerations**

Dermal adverse events are possible after the use of any topical product, especially in patients with pre-existing skin damage. Caution is required to avoid any contact with mucous membranes, especially with eyes. Topical insecticides should not be used on broken or secondarily infected skin. Chemical treatments should be used in children under 6 months only under medical supervision.

Aerosol-conditioning pediculicides are contra-indicated for people suffering from asthma, as cases of severe bronchospasms were reported [10]. If an aerosol must be used, spraying must be done in a well-ventilated room, preferably in the open air, avoiding misting in the direction of the eyes, nose and mouth. In most western countries, the propellant gas present in the aerosols is non-explosive and non-inflammable.

Preparations with an alcoholic base are not recommended for pediculosis with asthma, with scalp dermatitis (like severe eczema) or in very young children (under 5 years of age).

Chemical insecticides, especially alcoholic-based formulations can be a fire hazard, and burns have been reported. Application should be done well away from sources of flames and heat. Lastly, a recent case-control study suggested a significant association between childhood acute leukaemia and insecticide shampoos used for pediculosis. Even if causality was not formally demonstrated, these results need to be further investigated and may raise concerns by clinicians and families [11].

■ **Natural pyrethrins and synthetic pyrethroids**

Natural pyrethrins or synthetic pyrethroids have a low acute toxicity and a low occurrence of adverse events. Adverse events are most commonly dermal, with pruritus and rash being the most common findings. Rare cases of asthma exacerbations and even death have been reported in individuals after using pyrethrin-based products. Pyrethroid based preparations are contra-indicated in persons with an allergy to chrysanthemum flowers, as these flowers contain a natural pyrethroid.

Piperonyl butoxide has negligible acute toxicity and is not considered to have carcinogenic, teratogenic or genotoxic effects of significance to humans. Overall, natural pyrethrins or synthetic pyrethroids are recognised as having a good safety profile.

■ **Malathion**

There is no evidence to suggest that serious systemic adverse reactions are associated with topical malathion. Malathion has a relatively low acute toxicity by itself, but impurities, including isomalathion, malaoxon and trialkyl phosphorothioates, can increase the toxicity of malathion, as well as being toxic themselves. It cannot be excluded that scalp irritation may be caused by malathion but it is likely that some cases are due to the terpenoid vehicle used.

Systemic exposure to malathion after dermal application is low and below the oral acceptable daily intake of 0.2 mg/kg/day. With respect to any malathion that is absorbed, it is rapidly metabolised by tissue A-esterases and carboxylesterases to inactive metabolites that are subsequently excreted in the urine.

One case of miscarriage was reported to the Australian Adverse Drug Reactions Advisory Committee after use of a malathion head lice product, which was classed as possibly related to use of the product [13].

The available evidence suggests there are no new or significant safety concerns with malathion head lice products if applied in accordance with the instructions for use. Malathion should not be used for children under 6 months.

Reports of accidental ingestion of malathion are rare, as an extremely unpleasant odor would seem to deter ingestion. In the United States of America, between 1998 and 2003, the Toxic Exposure Surveillance System (TESS) reported 857 symptomatic cases of unintentional lindane ingestion. None of the cases were reported as resulting in death. Symptoms included vomiting (59%), nausea (18%), oral irritation (19%), abdominal cramping (4%), cough (4%) and seizure (3%). TESS also identified 523 symptomatic cases of unintentional ingestion of pyrethrin/piperonyl butoxide, permethrin or malathion (<50 cases). Among TESS reports, unintentional lindane ingestions were more likely to produce illness (857 illnesses of 1,463 ingestions [58%]) than all three of those medications combined (523 illnesses of 1,691 ingestions [31%]; odds ratio = 3.16, 95% confidence interval = 2.72-3.67) [12].

6.2.6. Which insecticide should we choose?

Various treatments are used as topical pediculicides worldwide but there is no clear consensus to define the best treatment for eradication of head lice. Following the recent withdrawal of a Cochrane review detailing available evidence, only a systematic review, published in 1995, is available. That review included seven randomised trials judged as unlikely to be biased. It concluded that sufficient evidence of efficacy existed only for 1% permethrin, with a lower 95% confidence limit of cure rate above 90%. Lindane and natural pyrethrins were less active while activity of carbaryl and malathion remained to be confirmed [7]. However, in the last 15 years since publication of this review, more and more reports have been published regarding resistance to pyrethroids and malathion, limiting its interpretation. Table 6.3 details recent evidence on the efficacy of chemical treatments.

In 1994, a French controlled study in schoolchildren showed that malathion was significantly more effective than d-phenothrin in both the clinical trial and *ex vivo* pediculicidal tests, confirming evidence of head lice resistance to pyrethroids in

Formulation tested	Agent in comparison group	Primary outcome	Result (tested formulation)	Result (comparison)	Ref.
0.3% d-phenothrin lotion	0.5% malathion	Lice eradication at 1 day Lice-free at 7 days	40% (39/98) (95% CI: 30-50%) 39% (38/98) (95% CI: 29-48%)	92% (87/95) (95% CI: 86-97%) 95% (90/95) (95% CI: 90-99%)	[8]
0.5% phenothrin	4% dimeticone, 2 applications 7 days apart	No evidence of head lice after second application or re-infestation after cure	75% (94/125) (95% CI:68-83%)	70% 89/127) (95% CI: 62-78%)	[9]
1% permethrin cream rinse applied for 10 min, twice at 10-day interval	0.5% malathion	Lice-free at 7 days Lice-free at 14 days	59% (13/22) (95% CI:39-80%) 55% (12/22) (95% CI: 34-75%)	81% (33/41) (95% CI: 68-93%) 98% (40/41) (95% CI:93-100%)	[5]

Table 6.3: Selected recent comparative trials concerning efficacy of pediculides with neurotoxic mode of action.

the studied population [8]. Since then, resistance to pyrethrins and pyrethroids has been reported worldwide (☞ Chapter 6.4.).

Today, chemical insecticides are often recommended as first-line treatment by national institutions. If a conventional insecticidal treatment for head lice infestation is chosen, it should be synthetic pyrethroids, synergised pyrethrins, or malathion. Indeed, the evidence on the efficacy of these products is based on published results of *ex vivo* and clinical trials. Nevertheless, therapeutic strategies may evolve with emergence of insecticide resistance. Resistance to pyrethrins and/or malathion raise concerns about environmental safety or long-term toxicity of chemical pediculicides and point out the need for development of alternatives to classical pediculicidal agents. Another major concern is the therapeutic strategy for difficult-to-treat patients (i.e., patients whose conventional treatments are ineffective, contraindicated or poorly tolerated) where traditional approaches have been unsuccessful.

6.2.7. References

1. Priestley CM, Burgess IF, Williamson EM. Lethality of essential oil constituents towards the human louse, *Pediculus humanus,* and its eggs. Fitoterapia 2006;77:303-309.

2. Clore ER, Longyear LA. A comparative study of seven pediculicides and their packaged nit removal combs. J Pediatr Health Care 1993;7:55-60.

3. Burgess IF, Brown CM, Peock S, Kaufman J. Head lice resistant to pyrethroid insecticides in Britain. BMJ 1995; 311:752.

4. Meinking TL, Serrano L, Hard B, Entzel P, Lemard G, Rivera E, Villar ME. Comparative *in vitro* pediculicidal efficacy of treatments in a resistant head lice population in the United States. Arch Dermatol 2002;138:220-225.

5. Meinking TL, Vicaria M, Eyerdam DH, Villar ME, Reyna S, Suarez G. Efficacy of a reduced application time of Ovide lotion (0.5% malathion) compared to Nix creme rinse (1% permethrin) for the treatment of head lice. Pediatr Dermatol 2004;21:670-674.

6. Meinking TL, Vicaria M, Eyerdam DH, Villar ME, Reyna S, Suarez G. A randomized, investigator-blinded, time-ranging study of the comparative efficacy of 0.5% malathion gel versus Ovide Lotion (0.5% malathion) or Nix Creme Rinse (1% permethrin) used as labeled, for the treatment of head lice. Pediatr Dermatol 2007;24: 405-411.

7. Van der Stichele RH, Dezeure EM, Bogaert MG. Systematic review of clinical efficacy of topical treatments for head lice. BMJ 1995;311:604-608.

8. Chosidow O, Chastang C, Brue C, Bouvet E, Izri M, Monteny N, Bastuji-Garin S, Rousset JJ, Revuz J. Controlled study of malathion and d-phenothrin lotions for *Pediculus humanus* var *capitis*-infested schoolchildren. Lancet 1994;344:1724-1727.

9. Burgess IF, Brown CM, Lee PN. Treatment of head louse infestation with 4% dimeticone lotion: randomised controlled equivalence trial. BMJ 2005;330:1423.

10 Chosidow O. Scabies and pediculosis. Lancet 2000; 355: 819-826.

11. Menegaux F, Baruchel A, Bertrand Y, Lescoeur B, Leverger G, Nelken B, Sommelet D, Hémon D, Clavel J. Household exposure to pesticides and risk of childhood acute leukaemia. Occup Environ Med 2006;63:131-134.

12. Centers for Disease Control and Prevention. Unintentional topical lindane ingestions - United States, 1998-2003. MMWR Morb Mortal Wkly Rep 2005;54: 533-535.

13. www.tga.gov.au/docs/pdf/headlice.pdf

6.3. Mechanisms of resistance

The fact that head lice may develop resistance to insecticides of any sort seems ostensibly unreasonable because in general terms it is known where all head lice live, on the heads of human beings, and elimination of these insects does not encounter problems of location, logistics and environment impact that would be encountered in eradication of, for example, mosquitoes that transmit malaria. The fact that head lice have developed resistance to several neurotoxic insecticides with different modes of action and that they continue to do so is not just a tribute to the adaptability and resilience of an apparently vulnerable insect, but also an indictment of human incompetence.

Simple survival of head lice after exposure to a chemical compound with pharmacological activity does not necessarily lead to resistance. The very fact that such an event has occurred means that it may recur and that some insects may acquire or develop a tolerance that can eventually render chemicals of that type ineffectual. When that tolerance is mediated by physiological mechanisms to detoxify or sequester the active chemical that would not normally be found in the insect it is reasonable to conclude that the insect has developed resistance.

Insecticides were first introduced primarily for control of clothing lice in order to prevent the transmission of typhus. The results, impressive at the time, were such that otherwise conservative investigators suggested that use of DDT might even have the capability to eliminate disease vector problems. However, it was not long before regular use of DDT for control of clothing lice on refugees and prisoners of war resulted in selection for resistant populations of insects. Reports of resistance began in 1952 amongst prisoners of war in Korea [1] and within a few years there was evidence of resistance to DDT from most countries in the world where it was in regular use. However, by that time, there was considerable investment for investigating more effective insecticides as a replacement because, apart from resistance issues, DDT was found not to be the effective panacea Buxton had anticipated. In fact it was slow acting, required relatively high dose levels, which despite the relative low cost of material made its practical use more expensive, and generally was not amenable to formulation in cosmetically acceptable delivery vehicles.

Remarkably, despite early recognition of resistance problems with use of DDT against clothing lice, no reports of resistance to DDT in head lice were forthcoming until the early 1970s, by which time the use of DDT was anachronistic in public health pest control in the developed world. By the time of these reports a putative resistance problem had already been identified with hexachlorocyclohexane (HCH or lindane), which had largely replaced DDT for most applications in the mid-1950s and had been investigated for control of head lice several years before that.

Reports of failure to cure using HCH became commonplace in London and parts of North East England by 1969 and an investigation of the problem suggested that resistance may have been the cause [2]. At that time lindane shampoo was the treatment of choice for most health practitioners and a major influence on the development of resistance would have been dilution in use of the product, particularly in areas where the tap water had a low calcium content, which meant smaller volumes of shampoo were required to achieve the same lather. It was shown that not only were head lice from the affected areas able to survive treatment with the shampoo they were also able to tolerate exposure to HCH treated filter papers in the laboratory. As a result an alternative insecticide from the organophosphorus group, malathion was introduced as a replacement [3]. However, re-examination of the data with hindsight raises some doubt about the conclusions of the investigations. No mechanism of action for resistance of head lice to HCH has been reported. However, in most developed countries alternative insecticides were introduced, partly in response to reports of suspected resistance and partly as a result of greater concerns about possible toxicological side effects of the use of this compound.

Alternative synthetic insecticides introduced in the 1970s included the organophosphate malathion, various pyrethroids such as bioallethrin, permethrin and phenothrin, and the carbamate carbaryl. In addition pyrethrum extract, a product derived from plants of the family Compositae, which had been used previously against clothing lice, was reintroduced for use against head lice. These chemicals were used, largely without reports of problems, from the 1970s through to the early 1990s.

Early in the 1990s crème rinse products containing 1% permethrin were introduced in many countries following several years of use in the USA and Canada. In most of these territories the products were so popular with consumers that they quickly acquired a majority market share. However, within 2-3 years cases of treatment failure were reported and when these were investigated it was discovered that the lice exhibited resistance both to permethrin and to related pyrethroid insecticides such as *d*-phenothrin. Resistance to phenothrin was first reported in France [5], followed by reports of permethrin resistance in Israel, Czech Republic, and the United Kingdom in the first instance, followed later by Argentina, the USA, Australia, and Denmark. Suspicions of resistance to these pyrethroids exist in most other developed countries and several developing countries.

Lice resistant to pyrethroids were quickly shown to be also resistant to DDT, suggesting a cross-over resistance was involved. "Knockdown" resistance (*kdr*), a point mutation in the *para*-type sodium channel gene that causes reduced neuronal sensitivity to the insecticide was identified as the most likely cause. In addition it was found that there were possibly contributions from detoxification mechanisms through elevated levels of enzymes such as glutathione S-transferase and monooxygenases but the contribution from these was not significant in lice from Israel [6]. However, lice from Buenos Aires in Argentina that exhibited cross-over resistance between permethrin, phenothrin, deltamethrin, and beta-cypermethrin, showed a significant increase of susceptibility to permethrin when treated simultaneously with the monooxygenase inhibitor piperonyl butoxide [7]. Some level of monooxygenase activity has been identified in several other isolates of resistant lice but in general the inclusion of piperonyl butoxide in treatment products along with permethrin is inappropriate because the primary degradation pathways for permethrin in most insects are via esterase activity. The lice from Buenos Aires also exhibited an increased susceptibility to permethrin when treated using triphenyl phosphate, an inhibitor of esterase enzymes, which indicates that resistance to permethrin operates via different physiological pathways in parallel [7].

Widespread use of permethrin continues so resistance to the insecticide is now also more widespread, although the intensity of resistance has probably reached a plateau in most affected areas. In most countries the identified cause of resistance is now confirmed as *kdr* and investigations have centred on the mutations involved.

Several studies have reported methodologies developed originally for investigating this mutation in houseflies in which the *para*-orthologous voltage sensitive sodium channel α-subunit cDNA fragments covering the IIS4 to IIS6 region were amplified by molecular cloning and sequencing. It was found that the most common point mutations were in the loci analogous to T921I and L932F in the IIS5 *trans*-membrane segment of cDNA [8-13].

Using cloning and sequencing of complete cDNA fragments additional mutations have been found in some isolates. Apart from the primary mutations (T917I and L920F in the numbering of amino acid sequence of the louse) an additional novel mutation M815I was identified in the IIS1-2 extracellular loop of the α-subunit from permethrin resistant lice from Florida, USA [9] and has since been found in 55/630 (8.7%) of the lice collected and was identified in insects from 11 of the 22 pre-

fectures of Japan [10]. The coinciding substitutions found in other, phenothrin resistant lice, from Japan were T951I and L955F, which were essentially the same as those from Florida lice, and an additional point mutation was identified at M850T [11]. A study in Denmark found that in addition to the two main mutations at T929I and L932F, one louse was found with a substitution at G943A in the *trans*-membrane segment IIS5 [13]. These sequence analyses show that head lice exhibit considerable variation in development of polymorphism in this segment of cDNA and that, although *kdr* overall may have had a common origin related to the relatively prolific use of DDT in the 1940s and 1950s, local variants have been selected spontaneously subsequent to the widespread introduction of pyrethroids.

What does this mean in practise for the harassed and busy parent trying to eliminate an infestation? Resistance due to *kdr* is a more subtle form of resistance than those mediated by enzymatic processes because the controlling gene is recessive and, as a result, a proportionality of approximately 1:2:1 is found in natural populations between homozygous susceptible, heterozygous resistant/susceptible, and homozygous resistant. Sensitivity to the insecticide is also mediated by factors such as initial concentration of insecticide, length of exposure, and bioavailability of the insecticide from the formulations as functions of the final dose delivered and the rate at which it reaches the target site. Thus heterozygous insects may prove to be susceptible to a given treatment if the dosing regimen is sufficiently intense, meaning that at least 75% of the insects may be killed. As most people use relatively inefficient methods for finding lice, it makes determining whether an infestation has been eliminated particularly difficult if only a small number of lice were present in the first place. Therefore, a low grade infestation may persist undetected after such a reduction in louse numbers and then when they have multiplied several weeks later to a number that is readily detectable by most people it is deemed that a new infestation has occurred. So far none of the mutations has been evaluated for the specific degree of insensitivity. It confers relative another mutation variant although all variants have been shown to confer around 3 or more times resistance compared with susceptible isolates [6-13]. In most cases it has also been possible to determine the LT_{50} (time to death of 50% of the lice) value for the insecticide exposure, which suggests that this form of resistance does not exclude killing the lice by normal therapeutic doses; it just makes it rather more difficult to achieve. However, where insecticide is detoxified or sequestered by either specific or non-specific enzymatic action there is a greater probability that lice may survive a treatment. No studies in head lice have actively investigated enzymatic degradation of pyrethroids, other than glutathione S-transferases and monoxygenases [6-8], but this pathway via esterase activity is likely to be more prevalent after a period in which lice with *kdr*-like mutations have been selected further by repeated exposures to ineffective treatments. In these circumstances the esterases active against organophosphate insecticides such as malathion would operate just as effectively against permethrin and phenothrin.

Resistance to pyrethroids has been of such impact that in several countries there has been renewed interest in the use of the acetylcholine esterase (AChE) inhibiting insecticides, mainly malathion. However, this also has suffered problems with resistance, with failures of treatment in France, the UK, Czech Republic, and Denmark. One possible cause is AChE polymorphism, with alternative, less insecticide sensitive, enzyme forms being selected when the primary form is rendered inactivated. It has been shown in susceptible body lice that there was a potential for a significantly higher transcriptional level for a paralogous AChE precursor compared with the orthologous AChE precursor, although this has not yet been confirmed to exert any advantage when challenged clinically with insecticide nor has it yet been demonstrated to be active in malathion resistant head lice [14].

Whether alternative AChE plays a significant role in malathion insensitivity may be somewhat academic as alternative forms of resistance may take precedence. Detoxification or sequestration of the insecticide by enzymes now probably plays the most significant role. Specific malathion carboxylesterase activity, detectable by synergising malathion with triphenylphosphate, was found to be 13.3 times greater in malathion insensitive lice from Bristol, UK, than in susceptible lice from Ecuador [15]. Similarly general esterase activity was found to be 3.9 times greater but there were no significant differences between the two isolates with respect to activities of phosphotriesterase, glutathione S-transferase, and acetylcholinesterase. It was found that the Bristol lice devoted a greater proportion of their metabolic output to producing esterases, with females showing 3.2 times the specific esterase activity compared with Ecuador lice and 1.6 times the protein content. Male Bristol lice showed 5.1 times the esterase activity and 1.3 times the protein content [15]. In this study the body weights of Bristol lice were not significantly different from those of Ecuador lice. However, in evaluations of malathion resistant lice from Cambridge, UK, it has been found that resistant lice are often considerably smaller than susceptible isolates, presumably because the insects have devoted so much of their metabolic output to enzyme production that their growth is retarded (IF Burgess, unpublished). Such activity presumably also crosses over to detoxify or sequester permethrin and other pyrethroids that are susceptible to this metabolic pathway.

In related studies it has been shown that isolates that were highly resistant to malathion also exhibited resistance to monoterpenoids incorporated into some medicinal products (e.g. Prioderm lotion, SSL International, UK; Ovide lotion, Taro Pharmaceuticals, USA) [16]. This means it is likely that most monoterpene extracts from essential oils, especially those that exhibit acetylcholine esterase inhibiting activity, have also been selected against and are detoxified by non-specific esterase activity. No doubt this has been partially selected for by the widespread use of essential oils in alternative treatments based on aromatherapy in which the materials are frequently diluted to sub-toxic levels. Resistance of this type is now likely to preclude from future use a wide range of compounds and plant extracts that have been considered virtually invulnerable by some sectors of consumers and have only recently entered into scientific assessments as possible pediculicides [17].

6.3.1. References

1. Hurlbut HS, Altman RM, Nibley C. DDT resistance in Korean body lice. Science 1952;115:11-12.

2. Maunder JW. Resistance to organochlorine insecticides in head lice, and trials using alternative compounds. Medical Off 1971;125:27-29.

3. Maunder JW. The use of malathion in the treatment of lousy children. Comm Med 1971;126:145-147.

4. Lamizana MT, Mouchet J. La pédiculose en milieu scolaire dans la région parisienne. Med Mal Infect 1976; 6:48-52.

5. Chosidow O, Chastang C, Brue C, Bouvet E, Izri M, Monteny N, Bastuji-Garin S, Rousset J-J, Revuz J. Controlled study of malathion and d-phenothrin lotions for *Pediculus humanus* var *capitis*-infested schoolchildren. Lancet 1994;344:1724-1727.

6. Hemingway J, Miller J, Mumcuoglu KY. Pyrethroid mechanisms in the head louse *Pediculus capitis* from Israel: implications for control. Med Vet Entomol 1999;13: 89-96.

7. Picollo MI, Vassena CV, Mougabure Cueto GA, Vernetti M, Zerba EN. Resistance to insecticides and effect of synergists on permethrin toxicity in *Pediculus capitis* (Anoplura: Pediculidae) from Buenos Aires. J Med Entomol 2000;37:721-725.

8. Lee SH, Yoon K-S, Williamson MS, Goodson SJ, Takano-Lee M, Edman JD, Devonshire AL, Clark JM. Molecular analysis of *kdr*-like resistance in permethrin-resistant strains of head lice, *Pediculus capitis*. Pestic Biochem Physiol 2000;66:130-143.

9. Lee SH, Gao J-R, Yoon K-S, Mumcuoglu KY, Taplin D, Edman JD, Takano-Lee M, Clark JM. Sodium channel mutations associated with knockdown resistance in the human head louse, *Pediculus capitis* (De Geer). Pestic Biochem Physiol 2003;75:79-91.

10. Kasai S, Ishii N, Natsuaki M, Fukutomi H, Komagata O, Kobayashi M, Tomita T. Prevalence of kdr-like mutations associated with pyrethroid resistance in human head louse populations in Japan. J Med Entomol 2009; 46:77-82.

11. Tomita T, Yaguchi N, Mihara M, Takahashi M, Agui N, Kasai S. Molecular analysis of a *para* sodium channel gene from pyrethroid-resistant head lice, *Pediculus humanus capitis* (Anoplura: Pediculidae). J Med Entomol 2003;40:468-474.

12. Kim HJ, Symington SB, Lee SH, Clark JM. Serial invasive signal amplification reaction for genotyping permethrin-resistant (*kdr*-like) human head lice, *Pediculus capitis*. Pestic Biochem Physiol 2004;80: 173-182.

13. Kristensen M. Identification of sodium channel mutations in human head louse (Anoplura: Pediculidae) from Denmark. J Med Entomol 2005; 42:826-829.

14. Lee S-W, Kasai S, Komagata O, Kobayashi M, Agui N, Kono Y, Tomita T. Molecular characterization of two acetylcholinesterase cDNAs in *Pediculus* human lice. J Med Entomol 2007;44:72-79.

15. Gao J-R, Yoon KS, Frisbie RK, Coles GC, Clark JM. Esterase-mediated malathion resistance in the human head louse, *Pediculus capitis* (Anoplura: Pediculidae). Pestic Biochem Physiol 2006;85:28-37.

16. Burgess IF, Lee PN, Matlock G. Randomised, controlled, assessor blind trial comparing 4% dimeticone lotion with 0.5% malathion liquid for head louse infestation. PLoS ONE 2(11):e1127.

17. Yang Y-C, Lee H-S, Clark JM, Ahn Y-J. Insecticidal activity of plant essential oils against *Pediculus humanus capitis* (anoplura: Pediculidae). J Med Entomol 2004;41: 699-704.

6.4. Resistance to chemical compounds

Several years after the description of resistance to DDT and lindane, other insecticides like pyrethroids or malathion started being widely used. As health workers and families began to notice difficulties of treating head-lice infestation, it was hypothesised that these pediculicides were becoming less active. In fact, studies of insecticides have reported treatment failure in laboratory bioassays and field trials. Before acquired resistance to insecticides is accepted as the cause of therapeutic failure, other possibilities should be considered but, as insecticide resistance is known to develop in insect populations where insecticides are heavily used, resistance to pyrethroids was suspected. D-phenotrin resistance was then first confirmed in 1994 by a randomised controlled study [1]. Since then, malathion and/or pyrethroids resistant-lice were observed in many countries.

6.4.1. Phenothrins

The hypothesis of d-phenothrin resistance was confirmed in 1994 by a controlled study comparing malathion and d-phenothrin lotions in French schoolchildren. Insecticides were administered under standard conditions, so that other possible causes of therapeutic failure were controlled for. Malathion was shown to be significantly more active than d-phenothrin in both the clinical trial and pediculicidal tests [1]. Since then, resistance to pyrethrins and pyrethroids has been reported by clinical and *in vitro* studies from a series of countries in Europe (United Kingdom [2], Denmark [3], Czech Republic [4]) as well as from Israel [5], the United States of America [6], Japan [7], Argentina [8] and Ecuador [9].

Resistance to pyrethroids and pyrethrins has been found to be associated with three-point mutations (M815I, T929I, and L932 F) in the voltage-gated sodium channel alpha-subunit in head lice [10, 11]. The three mutations are found together and probably coexist as a haplotype. Homozygous resistant and heterozygous lice are regarded as resistant to pyrethroids. The correlation between the resistant phenotype and the presence of this haplotype was confirmed in head lice from the United States [9], Denmark [3] and Japan [7]. This haplotype was also detected in Wales [12] and France [13].

A recent study confirmed the reliability and accuracy of a quantitative sequencing protocol that detects the frequencies of sodium channel mutations responsible for knockdown resistance in permethrin-resistant head lice as a population genotyping method. It is suggested that this protocol would be useful as a resistance monitoring tool [14].

6.4.2. Malathion

As expected, malathion resistance has been reported in many countries, such as United Kingdom [2], France [15], Australia [16], the United States of America and Denmark [3].

Head lice resistance to malathion could be associated with enzyme-mediated malathion-specific esterase mechanisms [17]. Evidence for double resistance to permethrin and malathion in head lice was reported in the United Kingdom [18] and in France [15]. Low levels of malathion resistance described worldwide suggests that malathion resistance in head lice is likely to expand with the increased use of malathion-containing products.

6.4.3. Conclusions

Pediculicide resistance is an increasing problem for the effective control of human head lice. Low level of resistance in some countries suggests that there is a high potential for head lice to develop insecticide resistance. Resistance to some pediculicides can vary from country to country and region to region within a country. Whether the findings on resistance can be applied to other parts of the world will depend largely on local patterns of insecticide usage. Clear treatment guidelines drawn up by healthcare professionals should take into account regional/national resistance patterns and propose evidence-based alternative treatments with no or low risk of development of resistance.

6.4.4. References

1. Chosidow O, Chastang C, Brue C, Bouvet E, Izri M, Monteny N, Bastuji-Garin S, Rousset JJ, Revuz J. Controlled study of malathion and d-phenothrin lotions for *Pediculus humanus* var *capitis*-infested schoolchildren. Lancet 1994;344:1724-1727.

2. Burgess IF, Brown CM, Peock S, Kaufman J. Head lice resistant to pyrethroid insecticides in Britain. BMJ 1995; 311:752.

3. Kristensen M, Knorr M, Rasmussen AM, Jespersen JB. Survey of permethrin and malathion resistance in human head lice populations from Denmark. J Med Entomol 2006;43:533-538.

4. Rupes V, Moravec J, Chmela J, Ledvinka J, Zelenkova J. A resistance of head lice *(Pediculus capitis)* to permethrin in Czech Republic. Cent Eur J Public Health 1995;3:30-32.

5. Mumcuoglu KY, Hemingway J, Miller J, Ioffe-Uspensky I, Klaus S, Ben-Ishai F, Galun R. Permethrin resistance in the head louse *Pediculus capitis* from Israel. Med Vet Entomol 1995;9:427-432.

6. Pollack RJ, Kiszewski A, Armstrong P, Hahn C, Wolfe N, Rahman HA, Laserson K, Telford SR 3rd, Spielman A. Differential permethrin susceptibility of head lice sampled in the United States and Borneo. Arch Pediatr Adolesc Med 1999;153:969-973.

7. Kasai S, Ishii N, Natsuaki M, Fukutomi H, Komagata O, Kobayashi M, Tomita T. Prevalence of kdr-like mutations associated with pyrethroid resistance in human head louse populations in Japan. J Med Entomol 2009; 46:77-82.

8. Picollo MI, Vassena CV, Mougabure Cueto GA, Vernetti M, Zerba EN. Resistance to insecticides and effect of synergists on permethrin toxicity in *Pediculus capitis* (Anoplura: Pediculidae) from Buenos Aires. J Med Entomol 2000;37:721-725.

9. Yoon KS, Gao JR, Lee SH, Clark JM, Brown L, Taplin D. Permethrin-resistant human head lice, *Pediculus capitis*, and their treatment. Arch Dermatol 2003;139:994-1000.

10. Lee SH, Yoon KS, Williamson MS, Goodson SJ, Takano-Lee M, Edman JD, Devonshire AL, Clark JM. Molecular analysis of kdr-like resistance in permethrin-resistant strains of head lice, *Pediculus capitis*. Pesticide Biochemistry and Physiology 2000; 6:130-143.

11. Lee SH, Gao JR, Yoon KS, Mumcuoglu KY, Taplin D, Edman JD, Takano-Lee M, Clark JM. Sodium channel mutations associated with knockdown resistance in the human head louse, *Pediculus capitis* (De Geer). Pestic Biochem Physiol 2003;75:79-91.

12. Thomas DR, McCarroll L, Roberts R, Karunaratne P, Roberts C, Casey D, Morgan S, Touhig K, Morgan J, Collins F, Hemingway J. Surveillance of insecticide resistance in head lice using biochemical and molecular methods. Arch Dis Child 2006;9:777-778.

13. Durand R, Millard B, Bouges-Michel C, Bruel C, Bouvresse S, Izri A. Detection of pyrethroid resistance gene in head lice in schoolchildren from Bobigny, France. J Med Entomol 2007;44:796-798.

14. Kwon DH, Yoon KS, Strycharz JP, Clark JM, Lee SH. Determination of permethrin resistance allele frequency of human head louse populations by quantitative sequencing. J Med Entomol 2008;45:912-920.

15. Izri MA, Briere C. First cases of resistance of *Pediculus capitis* Linne 1758 to malathion in France. Presse Med 1995;24:1444.

16. Hunter JA, Barker SC. Susceptibility of head lice *(Pediculus humanus capitis)* to pediculicides in Australia. Parasitol Res 2003;90:476-478.

17. Gao JR, Yoon KS, Frisbie RK, Coles GC, Clark JM. Esterase-mediated malathion resistance in the human head louse, *Pediculus capitis* (Anoplura: Pediculidae). Pestic Biochem Physiol 2006;85:28-37.

18. Downs AM, Stafford KA, Harvey I, Coles GC. Evidence for double resistance to permethrin and malathion in head lice. Br J Dermatol 1999;141:508-511.

6.5. Monitoring permethrin resistance in human head lice using knockdown resistance *(kdr)* gene mutations

Pyrethrins and pyrethroids have been widely used as over-the-counter (OTC) pediculicides. However, extensive use of these pediculicides, particularly permethrin, inevitably resulted in resistance problems (for details ☞ Chapters 6.3. and 6.4.). Permethrin resistance in head louse populations appears widespread worldwide but its intensity and distribution vary geographically [1], highlighting the necessity of proactive resistance management system prior to the complete saturation of resistance.

For the establishment of an effective resistance management system, understanding the molecular and genetic basis of resistance is imperative. Early studies by Clark's group demonstrated that knockdown resistance (kdr) is a major factor in all permethrin-resistant lice worldwide and supports the claim that treatment failure is largely due to resistance [2]. Three point mutations (M815I, T917I and L920F) in the voltage-sensitive sodium channel (VSSC) α-subunit gene identified in permethrin-resistant head lice were suggested to be responsible for kdr-type resistance [2-4].

Detection of the early phase of kdr is a crucial element in any long-term resistance management system designed to suppress resistance. Early resistance detection by conventional bioassay-based monitoring methods is very difficult, particularly when resistance is recessive. In addition, collecting large numbers of live specimens, as in the case of lice, is often impractical and difficult. To circumvent these limitations, various individual genotyping techniques for the detection of resistance allele frequencies and to determine allelic zygosities have been developed [5, 6]. In this chapter, we discuss on the current knowledge on molecular mechanisms of head louse resistance to permethrin due to kdr and the molecular techniques that can be used as alternatives for conventional bioassay-based resistance monitoring.

6.5.1. Molecular mechanisms of knockdown permethrin resistance

To elucidate the molecular mechanisms of permethrin resistance in the head louse, cDNA fragments that spanned the IIS4~IIS6 region of *para*-orthologous head louse voltage-sensitive sodium channel (VSSC) α-subunit gene were cloned and their sequences determined [2, 3, 7]. Sequence comparison between the permethrin-resistant and -susceptible strains identified three point mutations (M815I, T917I and L920F), all located in domain II, as putatively responsible for resistance (☞ Figure 6.4). All three mutations were determined to exist *en bloc* as a resistant haplotype through sequence analyses of cloned cDNA and genomic DNA fragments from individual louse samples, both containing the three mutation sites.

Functional analysis of the mutations was conducted by using the house fly *para*-orthologous VSSC α-subunit as a surrogate channel. The three mutations were introduced into the house fly VSSC α-subunit cDNA individually or in combination, and each channel variant was heterologously expressed in *Xenopus* oocytes [8]. Two-electrode voltage clamp analysis of the sodium channel variants with different combinations of the mutations revealed that the M815I and L920F mutations reduced permethrin sensitivity 2-3 fold when expressed alone but the T917I mutation, either alone or in combination, virtually abolished permethrin sensitivity. Thus, the T917I mutation plays a major role in permethrin resistance via a kdr-type nerve insensitivity mechanism, and can be used as a molecular marker for resistance detection.

6.5. Monitoring permethrin resistance in human head lice using knockdown resistance (kdr) gene mutations

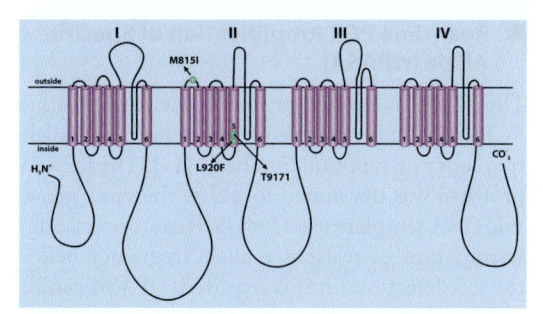

Figure 6.4: Transmembrane topology of the voltage-sensitive sodium channel (VSSC) α-subunit showing the location of the three mutations responsible for knockdown resistance (kdr) in the human head louse. Reproduced with permission from Ref. [14]. Copyright 2009 Elsevier Inc.

6.5.2. Molecular detection of *kdr* mutations for resistance monitoring

Various individual genotyping techniques for the detection of resistance allele frequencies using genomic DNA extracted from target insects have been employed as resistance monitoring tools [5, 6]. For the effective monitoring of head louse resistance based on the *kdr* genotype, we have developed three molecular techniques; (1) quantitative sequencing (**QS**), (2) real-time PCR amplification of specific allele (**rtPASA**) and, (3) serial invasive signal amplification reaction (**SISAR**).

■ **Quantitative Sequencing (QS)**

The QS protocol was developed as a population genotyping method for the prediction of *kdr* mutation frequencies (resistance allele frequency) in head louse populations [9]. Briefly, a 908-bp genomic DNA fragment of the VSSC α-subunit gene, encompassing the three mutation sites (M815I, T917I and L920F), was PCR-amplified from individual genomic DNAs (☞ Figure 6.5). After verification of genotype, the PCR products with opposite genotypes were mixed together to generate standard DNA mixture templates with resistant allele frequencies of 0, 10, 30, 50, 70, 90 and 100% and sequenced by cycle sequencing. The nucleotide signal intensities of both resistant and susceptible alleles at each mutation site were determined from the sequence chromatogram (☞ Figure 6.6a) and the signal ratios were calculated by dividing resistant nucleotide signal by the sum of the resistant and susceptible nucleotide signals. The signal ratios of template DNA mixtures were normalised by multiplying them with the normalisation factor (signal ratio of the heterozygous DNA template/signal ratio of the 5:5 standard DNA template). A plot of the normalised signal ratios versus corresponding resistance allele frequencies were produced and standard regression equations were created for the estimation of resistance allele frequencies of unknown samples and their prediction intervals at the 95% confidence level (☞ Figure 6.6b). Using the lower and upper 95% prediction equations, the average lower detection limits for the three mutations (M815I, T917I and L920F mutations) were determined as 7.4% at the 95% confidence level.

Since QS is designed to use genomic DNA extracted and prepared from multiple louse specimens, it is suitable for processing a large number of louse populations. The use of a single DNA extraction from multiple louse specimens greatly reduces the overall cost and effort as repetitive DNA extraction from individual lice is arduous and costly. QS for 90 different population samples can be completed within 2 days in moderately equipped laboratories. The technique dependency of QS is also

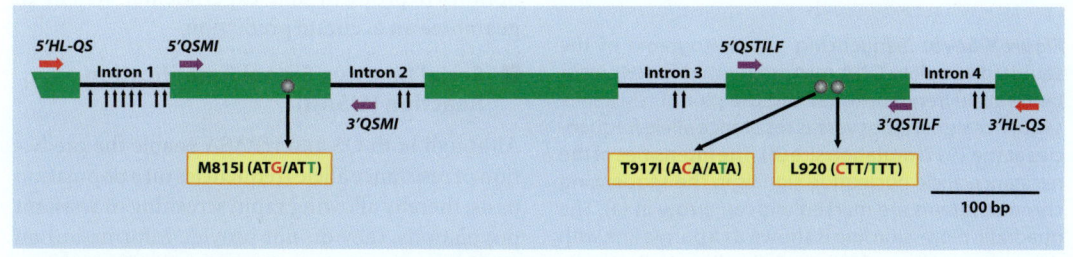

Figure 6.5: Exon-intron structure of the 908-bp head louse VSSC genomic region that contains the M815I, T917I and L920F mutations. Shaded boxes and solid lines indicate exons and introns, respectively. Locations of three resistance mutations are marked with black circles. Vertical arrows indicate the approximate locations of intron polymorphisms. Horizontal arrows indicate the locations of the QS primers. Reproduced with permission from Ref. [9]. Copyright 2009 Elsevier B.V.

relatively low compared to other population genotyping techniques such as rtPASA-TaqMan [10] and rtPASA. Thus, the speed, simplicity and moderate sensitivity of QS make it an ideal candidate for a routine primary resistance monitoring technique to screen a large number of field-collected louse populations as an alternative to conventional bioassay. Since the sensitivity of QS is ca. 7.4%, a small to medium-size sampling (7-14 lice) per louse population may be sufficient and is practical, considering the difficulty of collecting a large number of louse samples. Taken together, prediction of resistance allele frequency by QS will greatly facilitate the initial resistance monitoring efforts in field populations of lice.

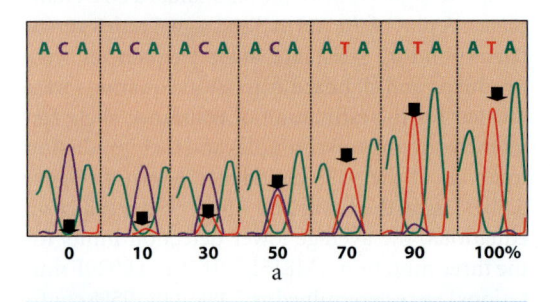

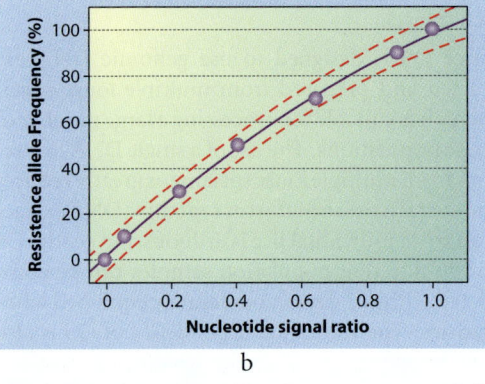

Figure 6.6a+b: Sequencing chromatograms of the standard template DNA mixtures with different resistance allele frequencies (a) and the plot of resistance sequence signal ratios versus resistance allele frequencies at the T917I mutation site (b). The intensities of the resistance allele nucleotide signals in the sequencing chromatograms are marked with an arrow in (a). The quadratic regression line is shown as a purple line with the upper and lower 95% prediction lines indicated by dashed red lines in (b). Reproduced with permission from Ref. [9]. Copyright 2008 Elsevier Inc.

■ Real-time PCR Amplification of Specific Allele (rtPASA)

The rtPASA is another protocol based on real-time PCR (rtPCR) for the prediction of resistance allele frequency on a population basis [11]. The rtPASA protocol was developed to utilise the same genomic DNA template used for QS. If more precise determination of resistance allele frequency below the QS detection limit is required, rtPASA can be employed as a supporting monitoring step. The standard DNA mixture templates for rtPASA were prepared as for QS except that different resistance allele frequencies were used (0, 1, 3, 8, and 16%). Allele-specific primers were designed to match the T917I and L920F mutation sites simultaneously (☞ Figure 6.7a). rtPCR was conducted with resistant allele-specific primer set using Chromo 4™ real-time detector (Bio-Rad, Hercules, CA), threshold cycle (Ct) values determined from each amplification curve, values normalised, and plotted against respective resistance allele frequencies (☞ Figure 6.7b). Standard linear regression lines for the prediction of resistance allele frequency were generated by plotting the log scale of resistance allele frequency versus Ct value (☞ Figure 6.7c). Once the prediction equation is generated, resistance allele frequencies of unknown louse populations were estimated by incorporating Ct values into the equation.

rtPASA enables the detection of the *kdr* allele frequency in the head lice at the level as low as 1.13%. To detect the resistance allele frequencies lower than ca. 1%, however, a large-size sampling (50~100 lice per population) would be required. In addition, the technical dependency of rtPASA is relatively high compared to QS, requiring a well optimised protocol and experimental system to guarantee an accurate prediction.

■ Serial Invasive Signal Amplification Reaction (SISAR)

Although both QS and rtPASA enable the prediction of resistance allele frequencies on a population basis, thereby allowing rapid screening of resistant populations, they do not provide information on allele zygosity (genotyping homozygous resistant RR, heterozygous RS and homozygous susceptible SS individuals). If information on resistance allele zygosity as well as allele frequency in a population is required, individual genotyping methods such as

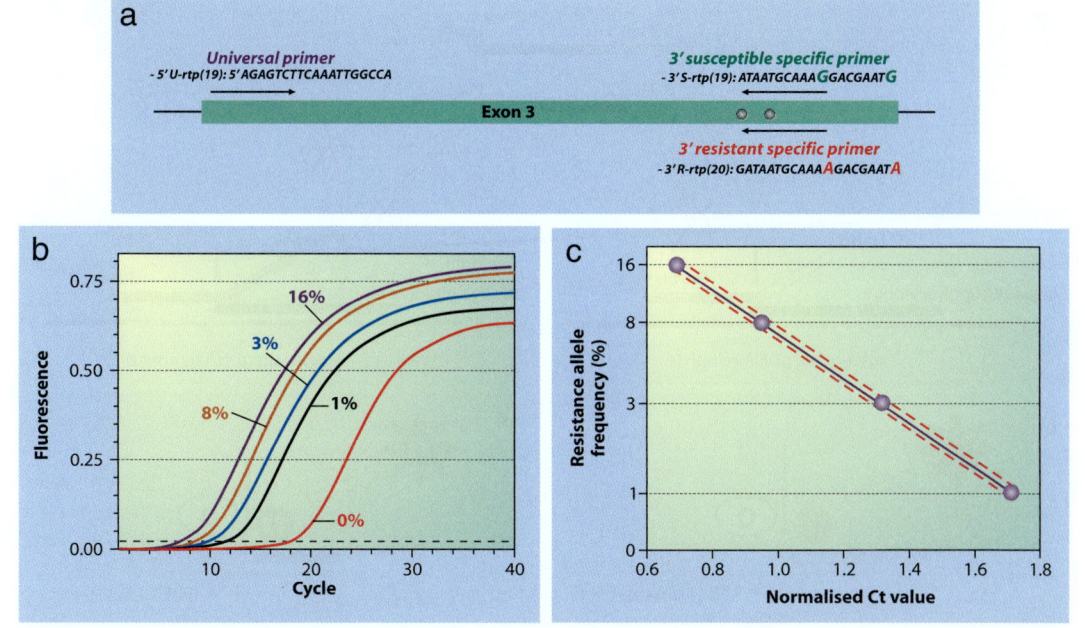

Figure 6.7a-c: rtPASA diagram (a), typical rtPCR amplification patterns using the DNA templates containing 0%, 1%, 3%, 8% and 16% resistant alleles (b) and the regression line generated from the plot of normalised Ct value versus the log of resistance allele frequency (c). Locations of the two mutations are marked with black circles and rtPASAprimers are indicated by horizontal arrows in (a). The regression line is indicated by a solid line with the upper and lower 95% prediction lines indicated by dotted lines in (c). Reproduced with permission from Ref. [11]. Copyright 2009 ACS.

SISAR [12] can be conducted on a much reduced number of populations as a secondary or tertiary resistance monitoring step.

The SISAR (☞ Figure 6.8) was originally developed for the high throughput analysis of single nucleotide polymorphisms using Cleavase®, a structure-specific endonuclease [13]. In the primary reaction, the invasive oligonucleotide anneals to both template DNAs. SNP-specific primary probes 1 or 2 anneal only to their complimentary template and the Cleavase enzyme cuts the 5' flap as indicated by the vertical arrows (☞ Figure 6.8a). The cleaved 5' flaps bind only to their complementary FRET cassettes and results in the specific cleavage of the fluorophore from the respective FRET cassette (☞ Figure 6.8b).

Information on allele zygosity is particularly useful for understanding the resistance population dynamics at the early stage of resistance where the resistance allele is present primarily as the heterozygous RS form in the population. SISAR requires, however, a large number of analyses (50~100 analyses of individual lice per population) to warrant accurate estimation of resistance allele frequency, which limits its applicability as a routine resistance monitoring technique.

6.5.3. Determination of *kdr* allele frequencies in human head louse populations worldwide

The three molecular techniques described above can be readily employed for routine resistance monitoring of head louse populations in a tiered system (☞ Figure 6.9). Although the proposed system only detects permethrin resistance mediated by sodium channel insensitivity, *kdr* is a major factor in all permethrin-resistant lice worldwide [2] and its detection should be useful for screening a large number of wild louse populations as alternatives to conventional bioassay.

Using these techniques, the resistance allele frequency and allelic zygosity of head louse populations collected from 14 countries worldwide were determined to construct a world *kdr* map (☞ Figure 6.10). Seven North American head louse populations were all collected from the U.S. The overall

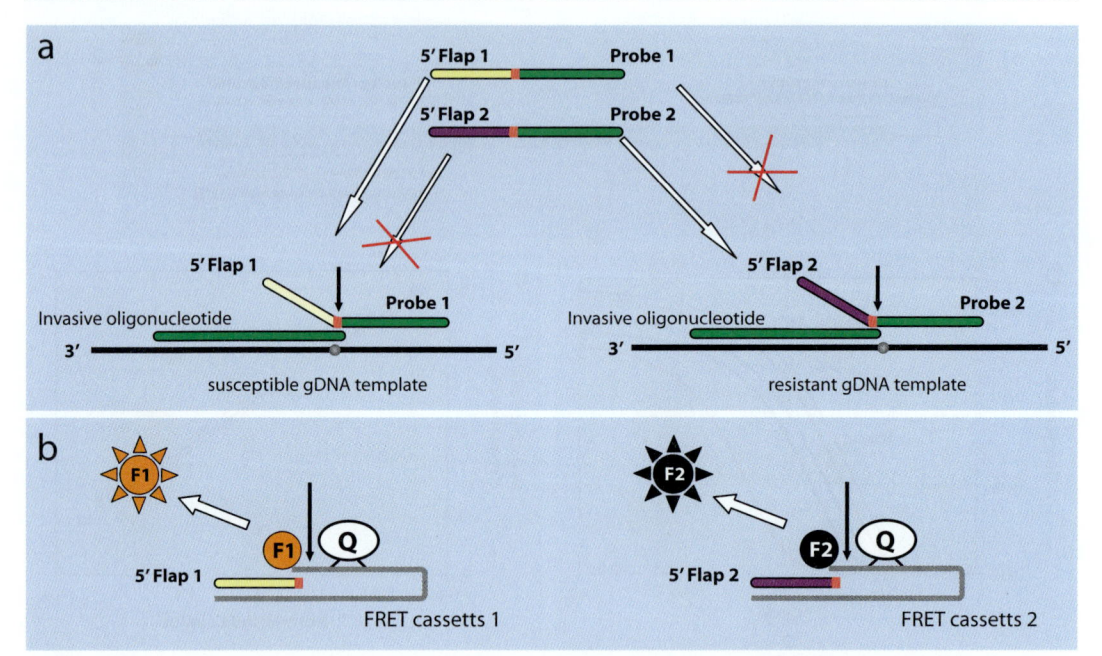

Figure 6.8a+b: Schematic of serial invasive signal amplification reaction (SISAR) based on matched enzyme (Cleavase)-substrate reactions. (a) is primary reaction. (b) is secondary reaction. Reproduced with permission from Ref. [12]. Copyright 2004 Elsevier.

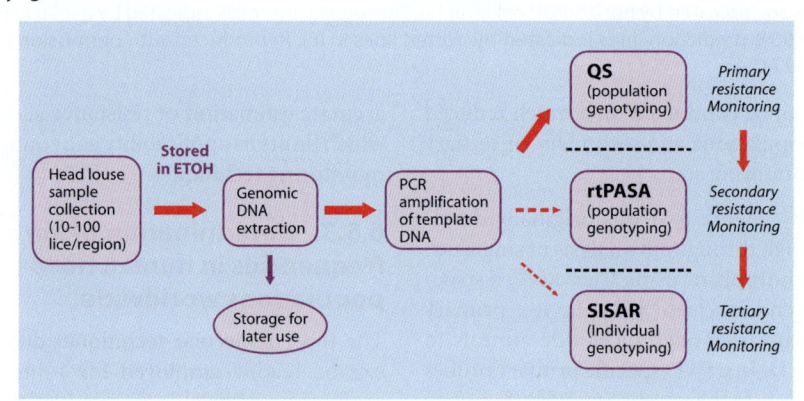

Figure 6.9: Tiered system for monitoring permethrin resistance in head louse populations based on several molecular tools. Reproduced with permission from Ref. [14]. Copyright 2009 Elsevier Inc.

allelic zygosities within the U.S. populations were 64.4% RR, 21.35% RS and 14.25% SS with a calculated resistance allele frequency of 75.1%.

In South America, five head louse populations were collected. Head louse populations from Argentina and Brazil had allelic zygosities of 86% RR, 7% RS, 7% SS; and 50% RR, 25% RS, 25% SS, respectively. The Ecuador population had 100% SS and the Uruguay population (n = 8) had 100% RR individuals. The calculated resistance allele frequencies were 89.5% for Argentina, 62.5% for Brazil, 0% for Ecuador, and 100% for Uruguay.

Three louse populations were collected within the European Union from the U.K., Denmark and the Czech Republic. Allelic zygosities were 100% RR in the U.K., 75% RR, 17% RS, 8% SS in Denmark, and 22% RR, 11% RS, and 67% SS in the Czech Republic. Based on their allelic zygosity values, the U.K. population had a resistance allele frequency of 100%, 83.3% in Denmark, and 27.5% in the Czech Republic.

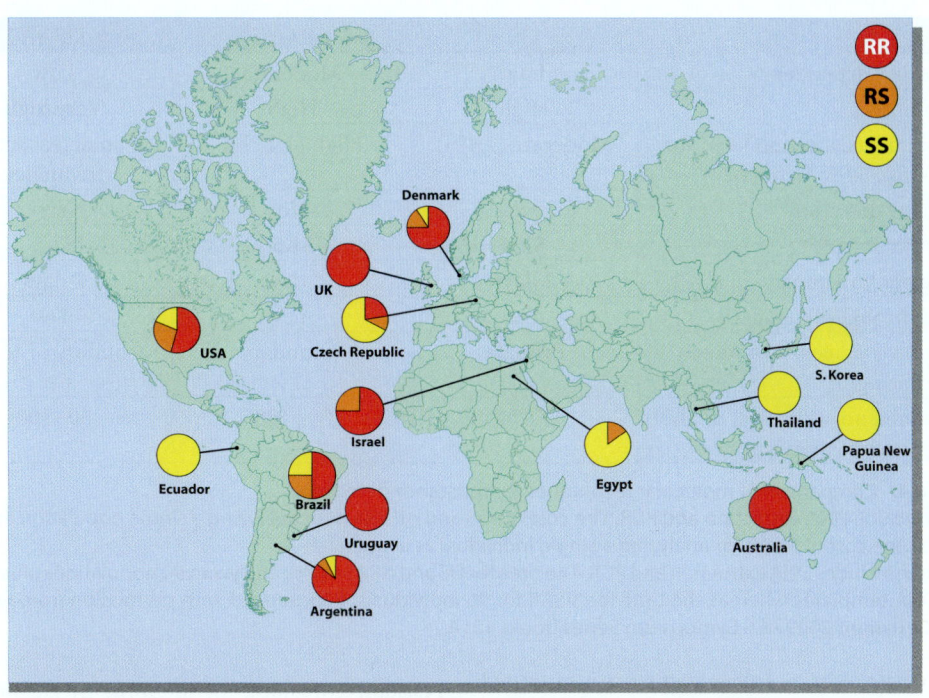

6.5. Monitoring permethrin resistance in human head lice using knockdown resistance *(kdr)* gene mutations

Figure 6.10: Worldwide occurance of permethrin resistant human head louse populations due to *kdr* mutations. Homozygous resistant populations (RR) are represented in red, homozygous susceptible populations (SS) are represented in yellow, and heterozygous populations (RS) are represented in orange.

No resistant homozygotes (RR) were identified in lice from Kafr-Elsheikh Governorate, Egypt. These lice only possessed 15% RS and 85% SS individuals, resulting in a resistance allele frequency of 7.5%.

No susceptible homozygote (SS) lice were identified from Israel. The allelic zygosity values of these lice were 75% RR and 25% RS, resulting in a resistance allele frequency of 87.5%.

All head lice collected from South Korea, Thailand, and Papua New Guinea were 100% SS. Comparatively, all head lice (n=28) collected from Australia were 100% RR.

6.5.4. Head louse resistance management

The three molecular techniques used to detect kdr in head lice were compared using the criteria of technical dependency, reliability, sensitivity, zygosity detection, cost, time, suggested usage in resistance monitoring and suggested number of lice per analysis (☞ Table 6.4). QS-based population genotyping can process a large number of louse populations simultaneously for the evaluation of resistance allele frequencies. Thus, the speed, simplicity and moderate sensitivity of QS make it an ideal candidate for a routine primary resistance monitoring technique to screen a large number of wild louse populations as an alternative to conventional bioassay. rtPASA can be employed as a secondary or supporting monitoring step. This method enabled the detection of the *kdr* allele frequency in the head lice at a level as low as 1.13%. If the information on resistance allele zygosity as well as allele frequency in a population is required, the individual genotyping methods, SISAR, can be conducted on a much reduced number of preselected populations as the secondary or tertiary resistance monitoring step.

In addition to detecting permethrin resistance mediated by kdr trait, accumulation of yearly and regional databases on resistance allele frequencies will greatly facilitate the monitoring and understanding of resistance evolution patterns in different geographical regions over time. Based on the resistance allele frequencies estimated by these molecular techniques, differential actions for resistance management can be implemented. In re-

	QS	rtPASA	SISAR
Technical dependency	Low	Moderate	Low
Reliability	High	High	Very high
Sensitivity (Detection limit for resistance allele frequency)	Moderate (7.4%)	High (1.12%)	Can detect actual frequency
Zygosity detection	No	No	Yes
Cost per sample[a]	$2.0	$1.5	$1.5
Time per 96 samples[b]	2 days	2 days	2 days
High throughput analysis	Yes	Yes	Yes
Suggested usage in resistance monitoring	Primary	Secondary	Secondary or tertiary
Suggested no. of lice per analysis for resistance monitoring	7~14	50~100	50~100

Table 6.4: Comparison of molecular techniques for resistance detection.
[a] Costs include DNA extraction and PCR. The cost for QS and rtPASA is for analyzing a single population as a unit whereas the cost of SISAR for analyzing a single individual as a unit.
[b] The time includes DNA extraction and PCR. The time for QS and rtPASA is for analyzing 90 populations plus 6 standard DNA templates whereas the time for SISAR for 96 individuals. Reproduced with permission from Ref. [15] 2009. Copyright 2009 ACS Symposium Series Books 1014.

gions where resistance allele frequency is saturated or near saturation, pyrethroids use should be curtailed and alternative pediculicides with different mode of actions used instead. In regions where the resistance allele frequencies are low or near zero, pyrethroids should be used cautiously and in conjunction with resistance monitoring program. This approach will extend the effective life span for this valuable group of pediculicides.

Recent completion of the human body louse (*P. corporis*) genome sequencing project allows us to acquire all the information on pediculicide target site genes and defense genes associated with pediculicide detoxification, and to use this information to effectively study resistance in the head louse. Interestingly, body lice have the smallest number of defense genes associated with metabolic resistance mechanisms (37 P450s, 12 GSTs, 18 Ests, 40 ABC transporters, etc.) among insects (Genbank www.ncbi.nlm.nih.gov/Taxonomy/Browser/wwwtax.cgi?id=121224). The small number of defense genes facilitates the construction of a minimal and efficient microarray for the identification and transcriptional profiling of a more complete set of genes that are differentially expressed in pesticide-resistant strains and involved in pediculicide-induced tolerance. The identification of such resistance mechanisms and novel target sites may allow the development of resistance-breaking compounds (e.g., negative cross-resistance compounds) for improved louse control, more inclusive molecular diagnostics for effective and affordable monitoring in resistance management, and specific non-toxic synergists useful in novel strategies to control pediculicide-resistant populations [15]. In addition to the aforementioned molecular techniques to detect the known mutations responsible for reduced sensitivity of pediculicide target sites, complete understanding of detoxification mechanism will enable to establish molecular methods to detect metabolic resistance as well.

Acknowledgements: This work was supported by the NIH/NIAID (R01 AI045062-04A3) and in part by the Brain Korea 21 Program.

6.5.5. References

1. Gao JR, Yoon KS, Lee SH, Takano-Lee M, Edman JD, Meinking TL, Taplin D, Clark JM. Increased frequency of the T929I and L932F mutations associated with knockdown resistance in permethrin-resistant populations of the human head louse, *Pediculus capitis*, from California, Florida, and Texas. Pestic Biochem Physiol 2003;77:115-124.

2. Lee SH, Yoon KS, Williamson MS, Goodson SJ, Takano-Lee M, Edman JD, Devonshire AL, Clark JM. Molecular analysis of *kdr*-like resistance in permethrin-

resistant strains of head lice, *Pediculus humanus capitis*. Pestic Biochem Physiol 2000;66:130-143.

3. Lee SH, Gao JR, Yoon KS, K, Mumcuoglu KY, Taplin D, Edman TL, Takano-Lee M, Clark JM. Sodium channel mutations associated with knockdown resistance in the human head louse, *Pediculus capitis* (De Geer). Pestic Biochem Physiol 2003;75:79-91.

4. Tomita T, Yaguchi N, Mihara M, Takahashi M, Agui N, Kasai S. Molecular analysis of a *para* sodium channel gene from pyrethroid-resistant head lice, *Pediculus humanus capitis* (Anoplura: Pediculidae), J Med Entomol 2003;40:468-474.

5. Clark JM, Lee SH, Kim HJ, Yoon KS, Zhang A. DNA-based genotyping techniques for the detection of point mutations associated with insecticide resistance in Colorado potato beetle *Leptinotarsa decemlineata*. Pest Manag Sci 2001;57:968-974.

6. Kim HJ, Hawthorne DJ, Peters TM, Dively GP, Clark JM. Application of DNA-based genotyping techniques for the detection of kdr-like pyrethroid resistance in field populations of Colorado potato beetle. Pestic Biochem Physiol 2005;81:85-96.

7. Lee SH, Smith TJ, Ingles PJ, Soderlund DM. Cloning and functional characterization of a putative sodium channel auxiliary subunit gene from the house fly (*Musca domestica*), Insect Biochem. Mol Biol 2000;30:479-487.

8. Yoon KS, Symington SB, Lee SH, Soderlund DM, Clark JM. Three mutations identified in the voltage-sensitive sodium channel a-subunit gene of permethrin-resistant human head lice reduce the permethrin sensitivity of house fly Vssc1 sodium channel expressed in *Xenopus* oocytes, Insect Biochem. Mol Biol 2008;38:296-306.

9. Kwon DH, Yoon KS, Strycharz JP, Clark JM, Lee SH. Determination of Permethrin Resistance Allele Frequency of Human Head Louse Populations by Quantitative Sequencing, J Med Entomol 2008;45:912-920.

10. Livak KJ. Allelic discrimination using fluorogenic probes and the 5' nuclease assay, Genet Anal 14. 1999; 14:143-149.

11. Lee SH, Clark JM, Yoon KS, Kwon DH, Hodgdon HE, Seong KM. Resistance management of the human head louse using molecular tools. In: Clark JM, Bloomquist JR, Kawada H, editors. Advances in human vector control. ACS Symposium Series, Vol. 1014. Washington DC: ACS Books; 2009. p. 203-216.

12. Kim HJ, Symington SB, Lee SH, Clark JM. Serial invasive signal amplification reaction for genotyping permethrin-resistant (*kdr*-like) human head lice, *Pediculus capitis*. Pestic Biochem Physiol 2004;80:173-182.

13. Hall JG, Eis PS, Law SM, Reynaldo LP, Prudent JR, Marshall DJ, Allawi HT, Mast AL, Dahlberg JE, Kwiatkowski RW, de Arruda M, Neri BP, Lyamichev VI. Sensitive detection of DNA polymorphisms by the serial invasive signal amplification reaction. Proc Natl Acad Sci USA 2000;97:8272-8277.

14. Lee SH, Clark JM, Ahn YJ, Lee WJ, Yoon KS, Kwon DH, Seong KM. Molecular mechanisms and monitoring of permethrin resistance in human head lice. Pestic Biochem Physiol 2010; in press. doi:10.1016/j.pestbp.2009.04.017

15. Clark JM, Lee SH, Yoon KS, Strycharz JP, Kwon DH. Human head lice: Status, control and resistance. In: Clark JM, Bloomquist JR, Kawada H, editors. Advances in human vector control. ACS Symposium Series, Vol. 1014. Washington DC: ACS Books; 2009. p 73-88.

6.6. Silicone oils for the treatment of head lice infestations

In the past few years, the most promising developments in the search for new effective compounds in the management of head lice infestations have been synthetic physically acting treatments, with silicone oils at the forefront [1].

The silicone oil dimeticone is used in different viscosities and concentrations in head lice products. Dimeticones (polydimethylsiloxanes) are synthetic silicone oils of low surface tension and can therefore coat most surfaces. These liquids consist of an inorganic silicon-oxygen backbone (…-Si-O-Si-O-Si-O-…) with methyl side groups attached to silicon atoms. The chain lengths of the polymers determine the molecular weight and viscosity, as well as the creeping and spreading properties. Silicone oils are commonly used in shampoos, conditioners, body lotions and similar products [2]. Oral dimeticones are also used as anti-flatulents to alleviate gastro-intestinal discomfort in postoperative periods and intestinal infant colics. They are physiologically inert—after oral ingestion, they are not absorbed in the intestine or metabolised, but eliminated unaltered in the faeces. In the animal model, no teratogenic, genotoxic or carcinogenic effects were observed after topical and oral application. The oils do not have any skin irritating or sensitising properties, and topical use in humans can be considered as safe.

Dimeticone-based fluids form a new class of head lice products. The silicone oil coats the louse surface and enters the respiratory tract, thereby blocking spiracles and tracheae (☞ Figure 6.11) [1, 3]. Böckeler & Richling (2008) have shown that the high dimeticone concentrated product NYDA® was capable of entering the whole tracheal system, subsequently asphyxiating lice (☞ Figure 6.12) [3]. Burgess (2009) considered claims of death by asphyxiation as controversial when testing a product containing a low concentration of dimeticone (4% – Hedrin®) [1, 4], but both studies agreed that lice are killed by physical means. This is of outstanding importance, as due to this physical mode of action, no development of resistance is to be expected (☞ Chapters 6.3., 6.4. and 6.5. for details on resistance of head lice against chemical neurotoxic pediculicides).

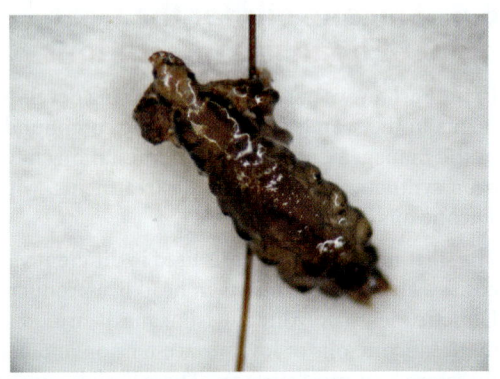

Figure 6.11: Head lice after application of a product containing a high concentration of dimeticone (Image: Jorg Heukelbach).

Several studies have shown the efficacy of products containing silicone oils as compared to neurotoxic insecticides [5-9]. An overview of available evidence of silicone oil-based products is given in Table 6.5. In general, these products are a safe and effective alternative for those patients who prefer not to use pediculicides with a neurotoxic mode of action.

Very high cure rates have been achieved with a high concentration dimeticone product. Heukelbach et al. (2008) studied 145 children and teenagers in a randomised comparative trial. After nine days, cure rate for patients treated with a product containing a concentration of dimeticone of 92% (NYDA®) was 97%, as compared to 68% for those treated with 1% permethrin [5]. In participants with heavy infestations (≥5 lice found at visual inspection before intervention), cure rates did not differ in the dimeticone group (97.1%), but decreased in the permethrin group (57.5%). At the end of the study, cosmetic acceptability was significantly better in the dimeticone group as compared to the permethrin group (p=0.01). The only product-related adverse event was mild ocular irritation after direct contact of the product with the eyes, which resolved quickly. In addition, the ovicidal efficacy of this product against young and mature eggs was shown in an *ex vivo* bioassay. After incubation of 60 minutes, efficacy (hatch rate of dimeticone group as compared to control group) against young eggs was 100%, and against mature eggs 95% [10]. Considering this clinically high efficacy and the excellent ovicidal efficacy, a single application may be considered as sufficient for management of head lice infestations.

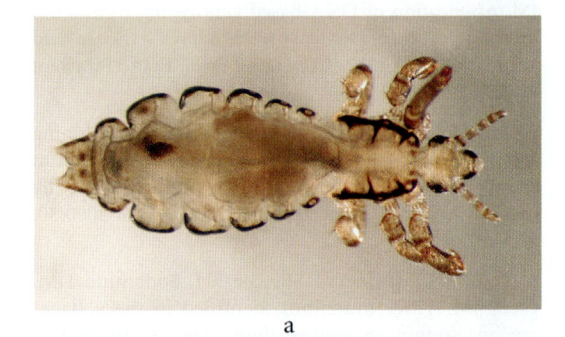

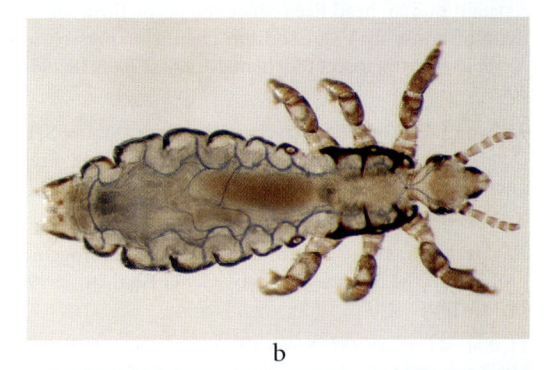

Figure 6.12a+b: A head louse before and after application of a blue-stained dimeticone solution (NYDA®). **a**: Air-filled tracheal system, slightly visible by total reflexion. **b**: Tracheal system filled with dimeticone solution. (Images: I. Richling & W. Böckeler, Germany; reproduced with permission).

6.6. Silicone oils for the treatment of head lice infestations

Product name(s)	Silicone oil	Other ingredients	Type of study	Primary outcome	Comments	Ref.
NYDA®	92% dimeticone (two different dimeticones of various viscosity)	Medium-chain triglycerides, jojoba wax, fragrances	• Randomised comparative trial (high concentrated dimeticone vs. 1% permethrin) • Comparative ex vivo studies on adult lice • Ex vivo ovicidal study	Cure rate 97.2% (NYDA®) vs. 67.6% (permethrin). 100% efficacy in both studies 100% efficacy (young eggs); 94.9% efficacy (mature eggs)	Itching reduced similarly in both groups. Better cosmetic acceptability of dimeticone product.	[5] [11, 12] [10, 13]
NYDA® sensitive	92% dimeticone (two different dimeticones of various viscosity)	Medium-chain triglycerides, jojoba wax	• Comparative ex vivo pediculicidal study	100% efficacy		[12]
Hedrin®, EtoPril®, Pouxit®, XTLuis®	4% dimeticone 96% cyclomethicone		• Randomised comparative trial (low concentrated dimeticone vs. 0.5% phenothrin) • Randomised comparative trial (low concentrated dimeticone vs. 0.5% malathion)	Cure rate 70% (Hedrin®) vs. 75% (phenothrin) Cure rate 76.9% (Hedrin®) vs. 34.5% (malathion).	No significant difference in cure rates. Significantly fewer irritant scalp reactions in dimeticone group.	[7] [6]
Full Marks® Solution, Resultz®	Cyclomethicone	50% isopropyl myristate (fatty acid ester)	• Randomised comparative trial (isopropyl myristate vs. 1% permethrin) • Randomised comparative trial (isopropyl myristate vs. 0.33% pyrethrum/4% piperonyl butoxide)	Cure rate 82.0% (Full Marks®) vs. 19.3% (permethrin) Cure rate 63.0% (Resultz®) vs. 22,2% (pyrethrum/piperonyl butoxide)	Low efficacy of permethrin due to resistant head lice. Interpretation of outcome limited, as treatment regimens were not standardised (second treatment after one or two weeks, according to infestation status).	[9] [8]

Table 6.5: Clinical and *ex vivo* evidence of head lice products containing silicone oils for which data are available.

6.6.1. References

1. Burgess IF. Current treatments for pediculosis capitis. Curr Opin Infect Dis 2009;22:131-136.

2. Yahagi K. Silicones as conditoning agents in shampoos. J Soci Cosmet Chem 1992;43:275-284.

3. Richling I, Böckeler W. Lethal Effects of Treatment with a Special Dimeticone Formula on Head Lice and House Crickets (Orthoptera, Ensifera: *Acheta domestica* and Anoplura, Phthiraptera: *Pediculus humanus*). Arzneimittelforschung 2008;58:248-254.

4. Burgess IF. The mode of action of dimeticone 4% lotion against head lice, Pediculus capitis. BMC Pharmacology 2009;9:3.

5. Heukelbach J, Pilger D, Oliveira FA, Khakban A, Ariza L, Feldmeier H. A highly efficacious pediculicide based on dimeticone: randomized observer blinded comparative trial. BMC Infectious Diseases 2008;8:115.

6. Burgess IF, Lee PN, Matlock G. Randomised, controlled, assessor blind trial comparing 4% dimeticone lotion with 0.5% malathion liquid for head louse infestation. PLoS ONE 2007;2:e1127.

7. Burgess IF, Brown CM, Lee PN. Treatment of head louse infestation with 4% dimeticone lotion: randomised controlled equivalence trial. BMJ 2005;330:1423.

8. Kaul N, Palma KG, Silagy SS, Goodman JJ, Toole J. North American efficacy and safety of a novel pediculicide rinse, isopropyl myristate 50% (Resultz). J Cutan Med Surg 2007;11:161-167.

9. Burgess IF, Lee PN, Brown CM. Randomised, controlled, parallel group clinical trials to evaluate the efficacy of isopropyl myristate/cyclomethicone solution against head lice. Pharm J 2008;280:371.

10. Heukelbach J, Sonnberg S, Mello I, Speare R, Oliveira FA. Ovicidal efficacy of high concentration dimeticone: new era of head lice treatment. Submitted. 2009.

11. Oliveira FA, Speare R, Heukelbach J. High *in vitro* efficacy of Nyda® L, a pediculicide containing dimeticone. J Eur Acad Dermatol Venereol 2007;21:1325-1329.

12. Heukelbach J, Asenov A, Liesenfeld O, Mirmohammadsadegh A, Oliveira FA. A new two-phase dimeticone pediculicide (Nyda sensitive) shows high efficacy in a comparative bioassay. BMC Dermatol 2009;9:12.

13. Sonnberg S, Oliveira FA, de Melo IL, de Melo Soares MM, Becher H, Heukelbach J. Ovicidal efficacy of over-the-counter head lice products (German). 104 Jahrestagung der Deutschen Gesellschaft für Kinder- und Jugendmedizin; Munich (Germany)2008.

6.7. "Natural" treatments and home remedies

Little is known about natural ectoparasite preparations used before the written word, however it is assumed that traditional, cultural approaches represent this oral lore. Written testimony to natural insecticides began in the first century AD when the Roman philosopher, Pliny the Elder, recorded known pest control methods. During the same period, the Chinese became avid users of powdered chrysanthemum, the forerunner of modern synthetic pyrethroid insecticides.

Before the introduction of modern synthetic insecticides, other so-called natural insecticides widely used for ectoparasites included pyrethrum (chrysanthemum), derris root, quassia, nicotine, hellebore, anabasine (tree tobacco), azadirachtin (neem tree), *d*-limonene, camphor and turpentine [1]. The chemical insecticide era began in 1939 with the discovery of dichlorodiphenyltrichlorohexane (DDT). Later organochlorines, organophosphates and finally synthetic pyrethroids followed. Such was the faith placed in these substances that natural product research significantly declined. Interest is slowly growing since resistance to many chemicals is increasing and becoming a global problem. Other relevant issues are the high cost of synthetic pyrethroids, environmental, occupational and food safety concerns, and the unacceptability and toxicity of many organophosphates and organochlorines. Despite this, many small and usually unfunded investigations have assessed potential bioinsecticides against a large number of pathogens and arthropods [2, 3].

Due to the failure of chemical insecticides to eradicate head lice, natural products for head lice proliferate with many street vendors offering their own concoctions promising total cures. It is commonly held that natural products kill lice differently from manufactured chemicals, but there is no evidence for this assertion due to the lack of an evidence base. Most insecticides function by targeting neurotransmitter receptors, ion channels and membrane transport processes, and researchers have not proposed that there are any new modes of action for natural products [4]. For example, pipronyl butoxide, a synergist, slows down pyrethrum biotransformation in insects in exactly the same way that the natural product neem does [5].

6.7. "Natural" treatments and home remedies

Also, the mode of action of pyrethrins is similar to that of organochlorines because both interfere with the permeability of sodium ion channels across nerve membranes. And further, the tea tree compounds 1,8-cineole and terpinen-4-ol act to inhibit acetyl cholinesterase as seen in organophosphate insecticides [6]. The difference is, though, that plants usually contain more than one active substance or synergists, thus reducing the risk of resistance.

Generally speaking, most insecticidal products derived from plants interfere with insect nervous systems and have very low mammalian toxicity. However they usually are quite toxic to non-mammals. Indeed, there are several organic phytochemicals of natural origin that are more toxic than some synthetic insecticides [7, 8]. Unfortunately, natural head lice products do not fall under the jurisdiction of therapeutic drug administration bodies and so their safety is not ascertained under the same stringent toxicological testing conditions required for manufactured chemicals [9, 10]. This is financially advantageous to companies marketing these products, but is detrimental to public safety.

A great deal of information abounds on the web and in books on herbal lore on how to use natural products to eliminate head lice. For instance, natural products such as olive oil are recommended to kill head lice, but in reality they only caused lice to go into stasis and recover fully after 5-15 minutes [11-13]. Thus, the information presented in this chapter is based on laboratory experiments and field trials rather than anecdotal and anthropological accounts and will focus on pyrethrum, tea tree and neem, among others.

Quite a few plants have been assessed in head lice bioassays and clinical trials, however, they are usually used in mixtures which makes it impossible to state which ingredient is the most active and what, if any, symbiotic or antagonistic action is present. The only generalised guidance was generated by a comprehensive *in vitro* study using body lice [14]. Twenty eight compounds were found in essential oils which were classified into high and low efficacy groups. Ono-oxygenated compounds and substances with flat compact molecules showed most activity. The top seven most active compounds had a methyl group.

6.7.1. Pyrethrins

Pyrethrins are bioinsecticides that are derived from extracts from the dried flower heads of *Chrysanthemum cinerariifolium* and *C. coccineum*. They have been tested more extensively than any other natural pediculicides. Clinical trials, including randomised comparative trials have tested the efficacy of pyrethrins in the field and have all concluded that they are very effective against susceptible lice [15-18].

Pyrethrins are still popular today, despite numerous synthetic analogues, because of several factors:
- they work well in certain situations
- they have a very low mammalian toxicity
- they rapidly biodegrade when exposed to UV
- they cause fast knockdown: the ability to rapidly render an insect unconscious on touch

Pyrethrins demonstrated efficacy in laboratory bioassays [19], and pyrethrum is often used as a control when screening potential bioinsecticides [15, 20, 21]. Unfortunately, resistance of head lice to pyrethrins in the field is common and up to an 80% decrease in susceptibility has been observed in the field in the last few years (R. Speare, pers. comm.).

Generally, mammals exposed to high doses of pyrethrin experience low reproductive effects, and no mutagenic or carcinogenic effects. Chronic exposure via a respiratory route can result in allergic responses that resolve after a few days. Natural pyrethrins vary in their acute toxicity and one should be cautious about inhalation, which can cause asthmatic attacks, respiratory distress, burning, itching and headaches. Severe poisoning may occur in infants who cannot physiologically detoxify themselves. The lowest lethal oral dose of pyrethrum is 750 mg/kg for children and 1,000 mg/kg for adults. Recovery from serious poisoning in mammals is fairly rapid [22].

6.7.2. Tea tree

Tea tree oil is steam-extracted from *Melaleuca alternifolia* and is comprised of over 100 hydrocarbons and terpenes [23]. Tea tree oil is commonly used in combination with other ingredients in natural pediculicides and pure tea tree oil has not been field evaluated in a formal setting. Only one clinical trial has evaluated tea tree oil in a mixture with

Carica papaya and thymol, a monoterpene phenol extracted from *Thymus vulgaris*. However, the evaluation criteria in this study were inadequately described [24].

Tea tree oil is less potent against head lice than pyrethrin but is still effective against susceptible populations [15]. Following exposure to a 1% tea tree oil emulsion, no mortality was observed for 2 hours, but exposure to a 10% emulsion caused 86% mortality [23]. A 4% tea tree oil emulsion mixed with 20% ethanol was observed to cause 100% mortality after four hours (J. Heukelbach, unpublished data). When the active ingredients were investigated, three likely candidates from tea tree oil (terpinen-4-ol, terralin and α-terpineol) were not effective at 1%, but caused 100% mortality at 10% [23]. Tea tree compounds 1,8-cineole and terpinen-4-ol inhibit acetyl cholinesterase in the same way that organophosphate insecticide function [6].

The topical use of tea tree oil in concentrations below 10% is considered safe because they usually do not cause irritant reactions [25, 26]. In one study on 160 patients exposed topically to a 5% tea tree oil lotion, 2.5% exhibited mild irritant reactions [27]. However, systemic hypersensitivity causing flush, pruritus, constricted throat and dizziness was recorded in response to a topical application of tea tree oil [28]. Children ingesting small amounts of 100% tea tree oil may show neurological signs, ataxia, decreasing responsiveness and even coma requiring assisted ventilation [29]. Recovery is uneventful and no deaths have been attributed to tea tree oil [26].

6.7.3. Neem

Neem oil is press-extracted from the seeds of the tree *Azadirachta indica*, (syn *Melia azedarach*) which is native to the Indian subcontinent, and is composed of triglycerides and triterpenoid compounds. One of the latter is a secondary metabolite called azadirachtin, a limonoid chemical compound belonging to the limonoids. Azadirachtin has toxic effects on insects, but is also an antifeedant and growth disruptor. Neem oil products have been extensively used as traditional Indian medicines for hundreds of years due to their insecticidal and repellent properties [30]. An open clinical trial using a shampoo containing neem oil dregs claimed that neem was highly efficacious, but the study design was not adequate which limits interpretation of results [31]. An *in vitro* trial using the same commercial neem product determined that it was far superior to permethrin [32]. In another laboratory trial, neem oil killed head lice slowly and was ineffective compared to malathion, permethrin and benzyl benzoate, but the units of concentration of active ingredient are not clear [33]. This study also reported that neem outperformed *Citrus medica*, and *Aloe vera* was completed ineffective. More recently, a well-designed *in vitro* study, that assessed mortality according to strict criteria, shed more light on the dose curve [34]. Extracts of ripe fruit (5-20%) caused 63-70% mortality while pressed oil (5-20%) caused 72-90% mortality. Combinations of the extract and oil with effective concentrations of 15-30% caused 86-97% mortality in exposed head lice.

The safety of neem has been assessed in many studies on acute and chronic toxicity and they all conclude that therapeutic topical use of neem is safe [30]. Oral ingestion of products containing neem, however, may cause intoxication and toxic effects [35]. Neem has the favourable qualities of being biodegradable and having a low mammalian toxicity, but is toxic to fish and other aquatic invertebrates [30].

6.7.4. Quassia

Quassia amara is known by several names and is famous for containing quassin, the bitterest substance found in nature [36]. Traditional uses include remedies for infestations of lice, helminths, anorexia and dyspepsia [37]. A topical scalp application of quassia tincture was used successfully to treat head lice in 454 patients with no adverse outcomes [38]. In an open clinical study, a quassia tincture had a 98% cure rate one week after a single treatment [39].

Quassia is considered safe by the Federal Drug Authority (FDA) since doses up to 1 g/kg do not cause acute toxicity in rats [40]. Parenteral administration, however, may cause cardiac irregularity, tremors and paralysis [41]. Oral ingestion of large amounts can irritate the stomach mucus membrane and may cause vomiting [41]. Excessive use may interfere with existing cardiac and anticoagulant regimens. The cytotoxic and emetic properties of the plant indicate that consumption during pregnancy is inadvisable [38].

6.7.5. Ylang ylang

A mixture of oils from coconut, anise and ylang ylang was evaluated in a field trial on primary school children [42]. The product was applied every five days in an unblinded comparative therapeutic trial with clearly defined assessments. The results were very good with the product effectively eliminating head lice infestations in 92% of study participants. A more recent randomised single blinded clinical trial compared the efficacy of a product containing coconut, anise and ylang ylang with permethrin lotion [43]. Efficacy of the natural product was significantly higher (82%), as compared to permethrin (42%). Interestingly, an *in vitro* study on ylang ylang did not show any significant effect on the survival of head lice [15], consistent with our studies in Australia that showed no killing effect against head lice *in vitro* (R. Speare, pers. comm.). Another study on coconut oil demonstrated its superior repellent properties [44], but it does not kill lice [45]. No papers have been published on the efficacy of anise alone.

6.7.6. Custard apple

Custard apple (*Annona squamosa*) has been highly efficacious in killing head lice in several studies [45-47]. The most recent study reported active components from *A. squamosa* seeds which tool between 30 and 62 min to cause 100% mortality according to the method developed by McCage [45]. In a small comparative trial on infested school children an extract of custard apple seeds in coconut oil killed 98% of head lice within two hours, and a petroleum ether extract of 20% *A. squamosa* seeds were observed to kill 95% of head lice three hours post product application. In these studies, seed extracts were more effective than leaf extracts [47].

Extracts of compounds in leaves and seeds from *A. squamosa* in petroleum ether, ether, chloroform and ethanol were tested for toxicity to the eyes and ear skin of rabbits [48]. Results on eyes and ears showed ether and petroleum ether to cause the most irritation and damage (conjunctival redness, chemosis, rugged cornea, skin erythema and oedema), while ethanol extracts caused mild eye irritation and no skin reaction.

6.7.7. Clove

The essential oils of clove buds and leaves have demonstrated activity against head lice comparable to pyrethrum [20]. This activity was attributed to the compounds eugenol and methyl salicylate which also displayed fumigant activity against head lice.

6.7.8. Lippia species

Essential oil from the African bush tea, *Lippia multiflora* at 25% concentration was found to be effective in combatting bodylice, head lice and scabies mites among Nigerian prison inmates [49]. It was more efficacious than benzyl benzoate, but was outperformed by kerosene.

In 2008 a patent describing the use of *Lippia javanica* was lodged [50]. It described the synergistic use of this species in a number of different formulations with other essential oils in killing ectoparasites and pests. Selected results follow:

- Formulation 1: 50% *L. javanica* essential oil and 50% carrier oil. Only 20% mortality after 60 minutes exposure.

- Formulation 2: Oils from lemongrass, rosemary (*Rosmarinum officinalis*), lavender (*Lavendula augustifolia*), tea tree (*Melaleuca alternifolia*) and red thyme (*Thymus vulgaris*). 80% dead after 60 minutes exposure and 100% mortality by 90 minutes.

- Formulations 3 and 4: Oils from *L. javanica*, lemongrass, rosemary, lavender, tea tree and red thyme. Instant knock-down and 100% mortality after 10 minutes.

- Formulation 5: Oils from lovage (*Levisticum officinalis*), marigold (*Tagete minuta*), lemongrass, lavender, tea tree and red thyme. 60% mortality after 60 minutes exposure and 100% mortality by 90 minutes.

Formulations that included *L. javanica* oil alone and those that did not include this oil failed to cause 100% lice mortality by 30 minutes. The addition of *L. javanica* essential oil to other essential oil compositions caused 100% mortality by 30 minutes and revealed a significant synergistic effect. *L. javanica* may thus prove to be a useful addition to the pediculicide arsenal [50].

6.7.9. Coconut

Besides the product containing coconut oil described previously (☞ "ylang ylang"), a recent clinical trial has shown efficacy of a coconut-derived shampoo [51]. Cure rate after 8 days was 61%, as compared to 14% in a permethrin control group. When all family members were treated, cure rate was increased to 96%. However, the pediculicidal action of coconut oil by itself is questionable. Lice reduce their activity after exposure to coconut, which enhances the effect to other ingredients.

6.7.10. Vegetable oils

Apparently lice can be killed by suffocation if heavy vegetable oils are used for a prolonged period. Oils from olives, soy, sunflowers, and corn have been observed to kill a "significant number of lice" if used in liberal quantities for more than 12 hours [52]. The low effectiveness of this method requires repeated treatments [52, 53]. Shorter exposure is ineffective as lice can render themselves impervious for over 20 minutes [11].

6.7.11. Eucalyptus and other herbs

Of several efficacious botanical essential oils identified by Yang et al., the most active was *Eucalyptus globulus* oil, followed by pennyroyal (*Mentha pulegium*), marjoram and rosemary oil which all displayed more activity than pyrethrum [15, 21, 54]. A recent study has shown efficacy of marjoram against lice that were resistant to malathion and permethrin [54]. Cade, cardamone ceylon, clove bud and leaf, coriander, cypress, *Eucalyptus citriodora*, myrtle, peppermint, spearmint, rosewood, basil and sage oil were also quite effective and showed similar activity to pyrethrum [15].

Unfortunately, some researchers have mistaken the physiological condition of stasis in lice, that occurs in response to encountering liquid [11] as equivalent to the knock-down effect observed in mosquitoes which can be fatal. For instance, in a fumigant knock-down test comparing essential oils and DDVP (2,2 dichlorovinyl dimethyl phosphate) against permethrin-resistant head lice, lavender had similar activity to DDVP, but eucalyptus outperformed both [55]. Another knockdown study in Argentina found a mixture of peppermint and eucalyptus oil to be as "toxic" as the best commercial product on the market [56]. Fumigant results alone are of no practical value in evaluating potential pediculicides.

In an earlier study conducted before basic standards had emerged in product efficacy testing, lice were immersed for 10 seconds in a solution and mortality observations were made 17 hours later with no interim blood meals provided [57]. A mix of red thyme and rosemary caused 87% mortality, and a mix of peppermint and nutmeg and another of tee tree and cinnamon caused 100% mortality. Leaving head lice without sustenance for 17 hours is not comparable to field conditions so these often cited results are of diminished practical use.

A well designed Korean study described a laboratory experiment that assessed the pediculicidal activity of *Cinnamomum zeylanicum* bark essential oil compounds against female head lice [58]. At a concentration of 0.25 mg/cm², the LT_{50} for this oil was 37.4 minutes compared to pyrethrum at 27.9 minutes. When the chemical constituents of the oil were identified and tested individually, the best performers and their LT_{50}s were: benzaldehyde (1.0 min), linalool (15.4 min), and salicylaldehyde (3.2 min). Fortunately, testing has shown that these three chemicals have low acute mammalian toxicity so their potential as pediculicides looks very promising [59].

Lastly, an *in vitro* study on 19 chemicals extracted from essential oils found a LT_{50} of around 25 minutes for (+)-terpinen-4-ol, (R)-(+)-pulegone, and 40 minutes for (−)-terpinen-4-ol and thymol. Results for the former substances are equivalent to those for pyrethrum and are promising [14].

6.7.12. Ovicides

While most commercially available topical treatments are effective in killing nymph and adult stages of head lice, they are ineffective in killing eggs despite their claims. This is because pediculicides do not penetrate the egg shell sufficiently to cause mortality and because they are mostly neurotoxic and the nervous system of a 1 to 2 day old embryo is too immature to be affected [60].

Veal's studies on ovicidal properties were interesting from a methodological viewpoint with several good results [57]. Lice eggs were exposed to a 1% concentration of each essential oil for 10 seconds (with either a water or ethanol solvent), shampooed and then rinsed in a 0.1% concentration with a vinegar/water carrier. They were placed in an incubator and observed until all the control eggs had hatched or died. In the ethanol solvent trial, rosemary and pine were completely ineffective, but tee tree, oregano, cinnamon, aniseed and red thyme caused 83-100% egg mortality. In the water solvent trial, only oregano and aniseed were effective and caused 99-100% mortality. In the Korean studies, cinnamon was observed to reduce hatching to 3% at 0.25 mg/cm² after 24 h of exposure. Component analysis showed no hatching with 0.063 mg/cm² salicylaldehyde, 0.125 mg/cm² benzaldehyde, 1.0 mg/cm² cinnamaldehyde and 1.0 mg/cm² benzyl cinnamate [58]. Marjoram was also shown to have an ovicidal effect with 58% of inhibition of egg hatching at a 1.0 mg/cm² [54].

Methyl salicylate and eugenol from *Eugenia caryophyllata* were highly effective at 0.25 and 1.0 mg/cm², respectively, but other test compounds and δ-phenothrin and pyrethrum showed little activity [20]. A subsequent study on *Eucalyptus globulus* leaf oil-derived monoterpenoids and terpenoids found that at 1.0 mg/cm², (–)-α-pinene, 2-β-pinene, and γ-terpinene exhibited moderate ovicidal activity, whereas little or no ovicidal activity was observed with the other chemicals, δ-phenothrin and pyrethrum. Ovicidal activity was dependent on compound and dose but the mode of action could not be determined [21].

And finally, in a study on 19 compounds found in essential oils evaluated at 1% concentration, few were found to have high ovicidal activity [14]. The best performers were nerolidol (70%), thymol (45%) and geraniol (42%).

6.7.13. Conclusions

Resistance to synthetic chemicals is not expected to decrease over time so expectations are high for natural alternatives. However, many natural chemicals with pediculicidal activity employ similar neurotoxic mechanisms to synthetic chemicals, which makes the search more difficult. Several of the botanicals and phytochemicals mentioned in this chapter have shown significant promise and merit further investigation. The number of methodologically meritorious clinical and *in vitro* investigations is lamentably insufficient so there is considerable room for future research. However, since head lice are not a major health concern, the burden of this research falls on entrepreneurs and commercial organisations interested in making a profit. While this sounds fine from an academic perspective, it has serious cost ramifications for the public. For instance, in the UK, quassia wood chips suitable for two treatments of long, thick hair may be purchased for around 2 euros. Unfortunately, manufacturers have made quassia prohibitively expensive in Australia where two treatments for long, thick hair cost AUD 64. When one is forced to pay this much for a product, quality control becomes a serious issue.

As with all grown products, environmental factors can greatly affect the quality and quantity of chemical constituents so strict standards are necessary for commercial production. The final issue of some significance to commercial operators is that of safety. Natural compounds are not subject to the same safety and quality standards to which synthetic chemicals are exposed. For this reason, safety data on many botanicals and phytochemicals are deficient and doses appropriate for safe human application are unknown. Future research should thus also include these aspects of quality and safety.

6.7.14. References

1. Compendium of Pesticide Common Names: Insecticides [http://www.alanwood.net/pesticides]

2. Roark RC: Some promising insecticidal plants. Econom Bot 1947;1:437-445.

3. Shaalan EA, Canyon D, Younes MW, Abdel-Wahab H, Mansour AH: A review of botanical phytochemicals with mosquitocidal potential. Env Int 2005;31:1149-1166.

4. Takano-Lee M, Yoon KS, Edman JD, Mullens BA, Clark JM: *In vivo* and *in vitro* rearing of *Pediculus humanus capitis* (Anoplura: Pediculidae). J Med Entomol 2003;40:628-635.

5. Andrews JR, Tonkin SL: Scabies and pediculosis in Tokelau Island children in New Zealand. J R Soc Health 1989;109:199-203.

6. Mills C, Cleary BJ, Gilmer JF, Walsh JJ: Inhibition of acetylcholinesterase by tea tree oil. J Pharm Pharmacol 2004;56:375-379.

7. Ciccia G, Coussio J, Mongelli E: Insecticidal activity against *Aedes aegypti* larvae of some medicinal South American plants. J Ethnopharmacol 2000;72:185-189.

8. Yang Y, Lee S, Lee H, Kim M, Lee S, Lee H: A piperidine amide extracted from *Piper longum* L. fruit shows activity against *Aedes aegypti* mosquito larvae. J Agric Food Chem 2002;50:3765-3767.

9. Sinniah B, Chandra S, Ramphal L, Senan P: Pediculosis among rural school children in Kelang, Selangor, Malaysia and their susceptibility to malathion, carbaryl, perigen and kerosene. J Royal Soc Health 1984;104:114-115, 118.

10. Jinadu MK: *Pediculus humanus capitis* among primary school children in Ife-Ife, Nigeria. J R Soc Health 1985;105:25-27.

11. Canyon DV, Speare R: Do head lice spread in swimming pools? Int J Dermatol 2007; 46:1211-1213.

12. Sinniah B, Sinniah D, Rajeswari B: Epidemiology and control of human head louse in Malaysia. Trop Geogr Med 1983;35:337-342.

13. Maunder J: An update on head lice. Health Visit 1993;66:317-318.

14. Priestley CM, Burgess IF, Williamson EM: Lethality of essential oil constituents towards the human louse, *Pediculus humanus*, and its eggs. Fitoterapia 2006;77: 303-309.

15. Yang YC, Lee HS, Clark JM, Ahn YJ: Insecticidal activity of plant essential oils against *Pediculus humanus capitis* (Anoplura: Pediculidae). J Med Entomol 2004; 41:699-704.

16. Casida JE: Pyrethrum flowers and pyrethroid insecticides. Environ Health Perspect 1980;34:189-202.

17. Stichele RHV, Dezeure EM, Bogaert MG: Systematic review of clinical efficacy of topical treatments for head lice. BMJ 1995;311:604-608.

18. Dodd C: Treatment of head lice. BMJ 2001;323:1084.

19. Taplin D, Meinking TL: Pyrethrins and pyrethroids for the treatment of scabies and pediculosis. Semin Dermatol 1987;6:125-135.

20. Yang YC, Lee SH, Lee WJ, Choi DH, Ahn YJ: Ovicidal and adulticidal effects of *Eugenia caryophyllata* bud and leaf oil compounds on *Pediculus capitis*. J Agric Food Chem 2003, 51(17):4884-4888.

21. Yang YC, Choi HY, Choi WS, Clark JM, Ahn YJ: Ovicidal and adulticidal activity of *Eucalyptus globulus* leaf oil terpenoids against *Pediculus humanus capitis* (Anoplura: Pediculidae). J Agric Food Chem 2004;52: 2507-2511.

22. OHS: Pyrethrum. In: Material Safety Data Sheet. New York: Occupational Health Services Inc.; 1987.

23. Downs AM, Stafford KA, Coles GC: Monoterpenoids and tetralin as pediculocides. Acta Derm Venereol 2000; 80:69-70.

24. McCage CM, Ward SM, Paling CA, Fisher DA, Flynn PJ, McLaughlin JL: Development of a paw paw herbal shampoo for the removal of head lice. Phytomed 2002;9: 743-748.

25. Crawford GH, Sciacca JR, James WD: Tea tree oil: cutaneous effects of the extracted oil of *Melaleuca alternifolia*. Dermatitis 2004;15:59-66.

26. Hammer KA: A review of the toxicity of *Melaleuca alternifolia* (tea tree) oil. Food Chem Toxicol 2006;44: 616-625.

27. Veien NK, Rosner K, Skovgaard GL: Is tea tree oil an important contact allergen? Contact Derm 2004; 50:378-379.

28. Mozelsio NB, Harris KE, McGrath KG, Grammer LC: Immediate systemic hypersensitivity reaction associated with topical application of Australian tea tree oil. Allergy Asthma Proc 2003;24:73-75.

29. Morris MC, Donoghue A, Markowitz JA, Osterhoudt KC: Ingestion of tea tree oil (Melaleuca oil) by a 4-year-old boy. Pediatr Emerg Care 2003;19:169-171.

30. Brahmachari G: Neem – an omnipotent plant: a retrospection. Chem Bio Chem 2004;5:408-421.

31. Abdel-Gaffar F, Semmler M: Efficacy of neem seed extract shampoo on head lice of naturally infected humans in Egypt. Parasitol Res 2007;100:329-332.

32. Heukelbach J, Oliveira FAS, Speare R: A new shampoo based on neem *(Azadirachta indica)* is highly effective against head lice in vitro. Parasitol Res 2006;99:353-356.

33. Morsy TA, el-Ela RG, Nasser MM, Khalaf SA, Mazyad SA: Evaluation of the in-vitro pediculicidal action of four known insecticides and three medicinal plant extracts. J Egypt Soc Parasitol 2000; 30:699-708.

34. Carpinella MC, Miranda M, Almiron WR, Ferrayoli CG, Almeida FL, Palacios SM: *In vitro* pediculicidal and ovicidal activity of an extract and oil from fruits of *Melia azedarach* L. J Am Acad Dermatol 2007;56:250-256.

35. Niemann L, Stinchcombe S, Hilbig V: Toxicity of neem to vertebrates and side effects on beneficial and other ecologically important non-target organisms. In: The neem tree – sources of unique products for integrated pest management, medicine, industry and other purposes. Edited by Schmutterer H. Mumbai: Neem Foundation; 2002:607-623.

36. Lewis WH, Elvin-Lewis MPF: Medical botany. Hoboken: Wiley; 2003.

37. Ninci ME: Prophylaxis and treatment of pediculosis [lice] with *Quassia amarga*. Rev Fac Cien Med Univ Nac Cordoba 1991;49:27-31.

38. Duke JA: Handbook of medicinal herbs. Boca Raton, FL: CRC Press; 1985.

39. Jensen O, Nielsen A, Bjerregaard P: Pediculosis capitis treated with quassia tincture. Acta Derm Venereol 1978;58:557-559.

40. McGuffin M, Hobbs C, Upton R, Goldberg A: American Herbal Products Association's botanical safety handbook. Boca Raton, FL: CRC Press; 1997.

41. Schulz V, Tyler VE: Rational phytotherapy: A physician's guide to herbal medicine. Berlin: Springer; 1998.

42. Mumcuoglu KY, Miller J, Zamir C, Zentner G, Helbin V, Ingber A: The in vivo pediculicidal efficacy of a natural remedy. Isr Med Assoc J 2002;4:790-793.

43. Burgess IF, Brunton ER, Burgess NA: Clinical trial showing superiority of a coconut and anise spray over permethrin 0.43% lotion for head louse infestation, ISRCTN96469780. Eur J Pediatr 2010;169:55-62.

44. Canyon DV, Speare R: A comparison of botanical and synthetic substances commonly used to prevent head lice *(Pediculus humanus* var. *capitis)* infestation. Int J Dermatol 2007;46:422-426.

45. Intaranongpai J, Chavasiri W, Gritsanapan W: Antihead lice effect of *Annona squamosa* seeds. Southeast Asian J Trop Med Pub Health 2006;37:532-535.

46. Puapatanakul A: A study on the use of seeds and leaves of sugar apple in treatment of pediculosis. J Pharm Assoc Thailand 1980;34:91-105.

47. Tiangda CH, Gritsanapan W, Sookvanichsilp N, Limchalearn A: Anti-headlice activity of a preparation of *Annona squamosa* seed extract. Southeast Asian J Trop Med Public Health 2000;31:174-177.

48. Sookvanichsilp N, Gritsanapan W, Somanabandhu A, Lekcharoen K, Tiankrop P: Toxicity testing of organic solvent extracts from *Annona squamosa:* Effects on rabbit eyes and ear skin. Phytother Res 2006;8:365-368.

49. Oladimeji FA, Orafidiya OO, Ogunniyi TA, Adewunmi TA: Pediculocidal and scabicidal properties of *Lippia multiflora* essential oil. J Ethnopharmacol 2000;72:305-311.

50. de Wolff R: Essential oil compositions for killing or repelling ectoparasites and pests and methods for use thereof. United States; 2008:1-54.

51. Connolly M, Stafford KA, Coles GC, Kennedy CT, Downs AM: Control of head lice with a coconut-derived emulsion shampoo. J Eur Acad Dermatol Venereol 2009; 23:67-69.

52. Meinking TL: Infestations. Curr Prob Dermatol 1999;11:73-120.

53. Mumcuoglu KY: Prevention and treatment of head lice in children. Paediatr Drugs 1999;1:211-218.

54. Yang YC, Lee SH, Clark JM, Ahn YJ: Ovicidal and adulticidal activities of *Origanum majorana* essential oil constituents against insecticide-susceptible and pyrethroid/malathion-resistant *Pediculus humanus capitis* (Anoplura: Pediculidae). J Agric Food Chem 2009;57: 2282-2287.

55. Toloza AC, Zygadlo J, Mougabure-Cueto G, Zerba E, Faillaci S, Picollo MI: The fumigant and repellent activity of aliphatic lactones against P*ediculus humanus capitis* (Anoplura: Pediculidae). Mem Inst Oswaldo Cruz 2006; 101:55-56.

56. Gonzalez Audino P, Vassena C, Zerba E, Picollo M: Effectiveness of lotions based on essential oils from aromatic plants against permethrin resistant *Pediculus humanus capitis.* Arch Dermatol Res 2007;299:389-392.

57. Veal L: The potential effectiveness of essential oils as a treatment for headlice, *Pediculus humanus capitis.* Complement Ther Nurs Midwifery 1996;2:97-101.

58. Yang YC, Lee HS, Lee SH, Clark JM, Ahn YJ: Ovicidal and adulticidal activities of *Cinnamomum zeylanicum* bark essential oil compounds and related compounds against *Pediculus humanus capitis* (Anoplura: Pediculicidae). Int J Parasitol 2005;35:1595-1600.

59. Budavari SB, O'Neil MJ, Smith A, Heckelman PE: The Merck Index. Rahway, NJ: Merck and Co; 1989.

60. Heukelbach J, Speare R, Canyon DV: Natural products and their application to the control of head lice: An evidence-based review. In: Chemistry of natural products: Recent trends & developments. Edited by Brahmachari G. Kerala, India: Research Signpost; 2006: 277-302.

6.8. Oral drugs for the treatment of head lice

Lice ingest orally administered compounds, when blood-feeding on their host. Consequently, several oral compounds have been tested regarding their efficacy against head lice infestation. The most promising drug is ivermectin. As oral drugs by definition are not efficacious against head louse eggs, a second dose after 8-10 days is generally recommended.

6.8.1. Ivermectin

Ivermectin is a semi-synthetic macrolytic lactone belonging to the class of avermectins. It was introduced for human use in 1981, in the first years almost exclusively for the treatment of river blindness (onchocerciasis). Since then, millions of individuals, mainly on the African continent, received the drug as a result of ongoing onchocerciasis and lymphatic filariasis control programs. Ivermectin is also highly efficacious against intestinal helminths and ectoparasites [1-3]. However, in many countries ivermectin is only approved for the treatment of certain nematode infections. As a result, off-label use for the treatment of ectoparasites, including pediculosis, is widespread. In fact, topical as well as oral ivermectin has been described in several trials as an effective treatment for pediculosis, with excellent cure rates [4-8]. The drug is very well tolerated, and adverse events are observed rarely. These may include fever, itching, dizziness, body pain and oedema, but are mostly mild and resolve within a few days. A single case of hepatitis following ivermectin therapy has been reported, but causality is doubtful, since the patient had been treated also with albendazole [9]. In fact, contrary to ivermectin, hepatitis is a well-documented adverse event of albendazole. Adverse events were not observed in patients who required repeated treatment with high dosages of ivermectin during a long period [10, 11].

In general, adverse events observed in patients with filariasis are related to the release of antigens from disintegrating microfilariae and not to the intrinsic toxicity of the drug [12]. So far, ivermectin is contraindicated for children younger than five years of age or less than 15 kg body weight because of the ongoing uncertainty of possible neurotoxicity of the drug and a less developed blood-brain barrier in small children. However, some data indicate that ivermectin is excellently tolerated also by children <5 years of age [13, 14].

In developing countries, particularly among resource-poor communities, people are frequently co-infected with various nematode and ectoparasite species. In these situations, ivermectin is an ideal drug for treatment of heavily affected individuals, and also for community-based mass treatment to reduce burden of a variety of parasitic diseases [1].

6.8.2. Trimethoprim-sulfamethoxazole (co-trimoxazole)

Co-trimoxazole, a mixture of the antibiotics sulfamethoxazole and trimethoprim, has first been suggested as a possible treatment for head lice infestation in 1978 by Shashindran et al. [15]. They had observed accidentally the pediculicidal effect of the antibiotic in a child treated with co-trimoxazole for respiratory infection, and subsequently performed a small trial on 20 individuals with head lice [15]. After oral application, lice were observed crawling to bed clothes and then dying. In fact, co-trimoxazole is not directly toxic to lice—the pediculicidal effect is believed to be a result of the antibiotic action of co-trimoxazole against bacterial endosymbionts living in the mycetomes of head lice, which the lice need for survival (☞ Chapter 6.11.). Endosymbiotic bacteria are transmitted transovarially and thus are passed from one louse generation to the other.

More recently, other authors reported that the use of combination of topical permethrin with oral co-trimoxazole would be an "emerging practice" in areas where head lice resistance is present [16]. Hipolito et al. (2001) observed promising results in a randomised three-armed controlled trial in children, comparing 1% permethrin crème rinse (cure rate after two weeks 79.5%) with oral co-trimoxazole (cure rate 83%) and co-trimoxazole in combination with 1% permethrin (cure rate 95%) [16]. However, cure was assessed by visual inspection, a rather insensitive diagnostic method, and information on outcome was partially obtained via telephone-based interviews of caregivers—a major drawback of this study. Sim et al. (2003) compared 1% lindane shampoo with 1% lindane + oral co-trimoxazole and obtained cure rates of 77% and 87% after two weeks, and of 91% and 98% after four weeks, respectively, but also did not use adequate outcome measures [17].

Independently from its efficacy, we do not recommend the widespread use of co-trimoxazole for head lice treatment, as there are other efficacious oral (ivermectin) and topical options available. An intensive use of co-trimoxazole for pediculosis would probably promote further bacterial resistance, reducing its value as an effective antibiotic drug. In addition, the compound may cause considerable adverse events such as nausea, vomiting, rash, pruritus and allergic reactions, and in rare cases agranulocytosis. Especially in countries where glucose 6-phospate-dehydrogenase deficiency is frequent, indiscriminate use of co-trimoxazole is problematic since it may cause severe haemolysis. However, the use of oral co-trimoxazole may be useful when head lice infestation is complicated by bacterial superinfection.

6.8.3. Albendazole

Albendazole (benzimidazole carbamate), approved for human use in 1983, is a potent anthelminthic drug used against many intestinal nematode and cestode infections. It is usually well tolerated by patients, and adverse events are rarely seen.

These may include epigastric pain, diarrhoea, nausea, vomiting, headache and dizziness. It is safe for use in children over 2 years of age.

A randomised five-armed trial reported some efficacy of oral albendazole against head lice [18]: One group received a single oral dose of 400 mg albendazole repeated after 7 days (cure rate after two weeks 62%), another group albendazole once daily for three days and after 7 days (cure rate 67%), the third group was treated with 1% topical permethrin (cure rate 80%), the fourth group received a combination of 1% permethrin and a single dose albendazole repeated after 7 days (cure rate 84.6%), and the last group 1% permethrin and albendazole once daily for three days and after 7 days (cure rate 82%). A fine toothed comb was also used in all groups as an adjunctive treatment. However, the outcome was not based on combing, but assessed by visual inspection. Additional studies are needed to conclude on the value of albendazole in head lice treatment.

6.8.4. Levamisole

Levamisole is an antagonist of nicotinic acetylcholine receptors occurring in the muscle cells of parasites. The compound is well-known as an effective drug against the human intestinal roundworm *Ascaris lumbricoides* [19]. There is one uncontrolled open study indicating that oral levamisole (3.5 mg/kg per day during 10 days) may have some degree of efficacy against head lice [20]. In this trial cure—defined as the absence of vital nits and lice—was observed in 67% of 27 participants after 10 days. However, due to the study design and inadequate outcome measure (visual inspection), interpretation of results is limited. Development of resistance of helminths to levamisole has repeatedly been reported [21].

6.8.5. Phenylbutazon

Phenylbutazon is a non-steroidal anti-inflammatory drug used for the treatment of ankylosing spondylitis. Its use is restricted almost exclusively to this indication, due to severe haematological adverse events, and the drug cannot be recommended for use in head lice infestation. Several historical studies, though, have reported a pediculicidal effect. A detailed review of available studies is given by Burgess (1995) [22].

6.8.6. Thiabendazole

Thiabendazole is a benzimidazole derivative with broad-spectrum anthelmintic activity. The substance binds to parasitic β-tubulin, and as a consequence inhibits microtubule polymerisation. Due to the availiability of the newer benzimidazoles mebendazole and albendazole, it is nowadays less commonly used. When given orally, adverse effects are more frequent than with albendazole and include anorexia, nausea, vomiting and dizziness; less frequent are pruritus, skin rashes, headache, tinnitus and hypotension.

An uncontrolled open study assessing the efficacy of oral thiabendazole (20 mg/kg twice per day, repeated after 10 days) in 23 girls with head lice concluded that this compound may be effective against pediculosis [23]. Visual inspection 10 days after treatment revealed a cure rate of 61%. Similar to the levamisole study, interpretation of results is limited, as an insensitive diagnostic tool was used to define infestation, and as there was no control group. Topical thiabendazole is effective against hookworm-related cutaneous larva migrans, but its value in head lice treatment is still not clear.

6.8.7. References

1. Heukelbach J, Winter B, Wilcke T, Muehlen M, Albrecht S, de Oliveira FA, et al. Selective mass treatment with ivermectin to control intestinal helminthiases and parasitic skin diseases in a severely affected population. Bull World Health Organ 2004;82:563-571.

2. Fox LM. Ivermectin: uses and impact 20 years on. Curr Opin Infect Dis 2006;19:588-593.

3. del Giudice P, Chosidow O, Caumes E. Ivermectin in dermatology. J Drugs Dermatol 2003;2:13-21.

4. Glaziou P, Nyguyen LN, Moulia-Pelat JP, Cartel JL, Martin PM. Efficacy of ivermectin for the treatment of head lice *(Pediculosis capitis)*. Trop Med Parasitol 1994; 45:253-254.

5. Youssef MY, Sadaka HA, Eissa MM, el-Ariny AF. Topical application of ivermectin for human ectoparasites. Am J Trop Med Hyg 1995;53:652-653.

6. Strycharz JP, Yoon KS, Clark JM. A new ivermectin formulation topically kills permethrin-resistant human head lice (Anoplura: Pediculidae). J Med Entomol 2008; 45:75-81.

7. Heukelbach J, Wilcke T, Winter B, Sales de Oliveira FA, Saboia Moura RC, Harms G, et al. Efficacy of ivermectin in a patient population concomitantly infected

with intestinal helminths and ectoparasites. Arzneimittelforschung 2004;54:416-421.

8. Dunne CL, Malone CJ, Whitworth JAG. A field study of the effects of ivermectin on ectoparasites of man. Trans R Soc Trop Med Hyg 1991;85:550-551.

9. Veit O, Beck B, Steuerwald M, Hatz C. First case of ivermectin-induced severe hepatitis. Trans R Soc Trop Med Hyg 2006;100:795-797.

10. Guzzo CA, Furtek CI, Porras AG, Chen C, Tipping R, Clineschmidt CM, et al. Safety, tolerability, and pharmacokinetics of escalating high doses of ivermectin in healthy adult subjects. J Clin Pharmacol 2002;42:1122-1133.

11. Richter J, Schwarz U, Duwe S, Ellerbrok H, Poggensee G, Pauli G. [Recurrent strongyloidiasis as an indicator of HTLV-1 infection]. Dtsch Med Wochenschr 2005; 130:1007-1010.

12. Kamgno J, Gardon J, Gardon-Wendel N, Demanga N, Duke BO, Boussinesq M. Adverse systemic reactions to treatment of onchocerciasis with ivermectin at normal and high doses given annually or three-monthly. Trans R Soc Trop Med Hyg 2004;98:496-504.

13. Brooks PA, Grace RF. Ivermectin is better than benzyl benzoate for childhood scabies in developing countries. J Pediatr Child Health 2002;38:401-404.

14. Sáez-de-Ocariz MM, McKinster CD, Orozco-Covarrubias L, Tamayo-Sánchez L, Ruiz-Maldonado R. Treatment of 18 children with scabies or cutaneous larva migrans using ivermectin. Clin Dermatol 2002;27:264-267.

15. Shashindran CH, Gandhi IS, Krishnasamy S, Ghosh MN. Oral therapy of pediculosis capitis with cotrimoxazole. Br J Dermatol 1978;98:699-700.

16. Hipolito RB, Mallorca FG, Zuniga-Macaraig ZO, Apolinario PC, Wheeler-Sherman J. Head lice infestation: single drug versus combination therapy with one percent permethrin and trimethoprim/sulfamethoxazole. Pediatrics 2001;107:E30.

17. Sim S, Lee IY, Lee KJ, Seo JH, Im KI, Shin MH, et al. A survey on head lice infestation in Korea (2001) and the therapeutic efficacy of oral trimethoprim/sulfamethoxazole adding to lindane shampoo. Korean J Parasitol 2003; 41:57-61.

18. Akisu C, Delibas SB, Aksoy U. Albendazole: single or combination therapy with permethrin against pediculosis capitis. Pediatr Dermatol 2006;23:179-182.

19. Keiser J, Utzinger J. Efficacy of current drugs against soil-transmitted helminth infections: systematic review and meta-analysis. JAMA 2008;299:1937-1948.

20. Namazi MR. Levamisole: a safe and economical weapon against pediculosis. Int J Dermatol 2001;40:292-294.

21. Martin RJ, Robertson AP. Mode of action of levamisole and pyrantel, anthelmintic resistance, E153 and Q57. Parasitology 2007; 34:1093-1104.

22. Burgess IF. Human lice and their management. Adv Parasitol 1995;36: 71-342.

23. Namazi MR. Treatment of pediculosis capitis with thiabendazole: a pilot study. Int J Dermatol 2003;42: 973-976.

6.9. Other approaches for head lice management: spinosad and oxyphthirine®

6.9.1. Spinosad

Spinosyns are macrolytic lactones. Spinosad is a mixture of two spinosyns, which are natural fermentation products of the actinomycete *Saccharopolyspora spinosa*. The aerobic gram-positive bacterium *S. spinosa* was first isolated by a pharmaceutical company from soil samples of an abandoned rum distillery on the Virgin Islands in 1983 [1]. In 1997, spinosad was launched as a commercial insecticide against caterpillars resistant to pyrethroids, and in the year 2000 the first veterinary product for use in sheep was marketed in Australia. Since then, spinosad has been used more and more for insect and ectoparasite control in veterinary medicine, and topical applications have shown a good efficacy against lice of livestock [2, 3]. Other applications include the management of pests in agriculture.

Spinosad's mode of action against insects is based on blocking of nicotinic acetylcholine and GABA receptors. As a consequence, insects are killed by hyperexcitation of the nervous system resulting in paralysis [4]. Spinosad has a very low mammalian toxicity.

Two published studies have shown a high *in vitro* efficacy of spinosad against permethrin-resistant head lice and also against head louse eggs [5, 6]. In addition, a patent application publication from the USA presents data on high ovicidal efficacy after immersion for 10 minutes in spinosad [7]: not a single egg hatched after treatment with 1% spinosad, as compared to 98% hatch rate in a control group exposed to water. In this report, pediculicidal efficacy was also high. Several phase III comparative trials have been undertaken by a pharmaceutical company in the USA, where it is planned to be marketed under the name NatrOVA™, but results have not yet been published in the scientific literature [8]. In conclusion, spinosad may be a new effective option for head lice therapy.

6.9.2. Oxyphthirine®

Oxyphthirine® is a compound based on triglycerides and lipid esters. Lice are claimed to be killed by asphyxiation, but no adequate laboratory-based or clinical data are published confirming this assumption. In one recent *ex vivo* assay, efficacy of an oxyphthirine®-product (Liberalice/DUO LP-PRO®) was low, indicating that a single topical application, as recommended by the producer, is not sufficient to eradicate lice [9].

6.9.3. References

1. Mertz FP, Yao RC. *Saccharopolyspora spinosa* sp. nov. isolated from soil collected in a sugar mill rum still. Int J Syst Bacteriol 1990;40:34-39.

2. Huang KX, Xia L, Zhang Y, Ding X, Zahn JA. Recent advances in the biochemistry of spinosyns. Appl Microbiol Biotechnol 2009;82:13-23.

3. White WH, Hutchens DE, Jones C, Firkins LD, Paul AJ, Smith LL, et al. Therapeutic and persistent efficacy of spinosad applied as a pour-on or a topical spray against natural infestations of chewing and sucking lice on cattle. Vet Parasitol 2007;143:329-336.

4. Salgado VL. Studies on the mode of action of spinosad: insect symptoms and physiological correlates. Pestic Biochem Physiol 1998;60:91-201.

5. Mougabure CG, Zerba EN, Picollo MI. Permethrin-resistant head lice (Anoplura: Pediculidae) in Argentina are susceptible to spinosad. J Med Entomol 2006;43:634-635.

6. Cueto GM, Zerba E, Picollo MI. Embryonic development of human lice: rearing conditions and susceptibility to spinosad. Mem Inst Oswaldo Cruz 2006;101:257-261.

7. Janssen H, Ho K, Nystrand G, Williams D, Lamb CS, inventors; Pediculicidal and ovacidal treatment compositions and methods for killing head lice and their eggs. Patent US2006/0024345 A1. United States of America 2006.

8. ParaProPharmaceuticals. A phase 3 comparative safety and efficacy study between NatrOVA creme rinse - 1% and NIX creme rinse in subjects >6 months of age or older with pediculosis capitis. Clinical Trial Identifier: NCT005457532008.

9. Heukelbach J, Asenov A, Liesenfeld O, Mirmohammadsadegh A, Oliveira FA. A new dimeticone pediculicide shows high efficacy in a comparative bioassay. BMC Dermatol 2009;9:12.

6.10. Head lice repellents

The failure of pediculicide products in many countries (☞ Chapter 6.4.) has resulted in increased consideration of preventative methods, which most commonly involve the use of repellents. In general, insect repellents are used as a means of personal protection against biting arthropods. At present, one of the most effective methodologies to prevent transmission of insect-borne disease is to use repellents, which over-sensitise the chemoreceptive organs of the vector and disorient it from seeking a blood meal from a human host. Lice repellents were thus initially drawn from the arsenal of chemicals commonly found to be effective against other insects such as mosquitoes and biting flies; however little empirical evidence exists. Herbal lore often promotes the use of essential oils, however, in most cases, little more than anecdotal evidence exists and empirical evidence does not tend to substantiate claims of efficacy or is contradictory. With increasing global prevalence of pediculosis and accompanying increasing awareness, the number of head lice repellents and preventatives available over the counter has increased dramatically without any quality assurance or control. Although synthetic chemicals require scrutiny before they reach the market, botanical formulations and phytochemicals require no testing for either efficacy or toxicity.

6.10.1. Repellent mechanisms

The purpose of a repellent is simple: It aims to drive away or ward off a targeted pest. The mechanisms are diverse. Some impose a mechanical barrier, some elicit a response from receptors, which translate to aversion due to any number of unknown reasons that may range from disgust to distain, some mask host emanations and others disrupt receptor function.

The few available studies on lice repellents fail in that they do not present a complete picture of repellence and focus only on avoidance. Since repellence is caused by so many different mechanisms, and head lice move readily between heads [1], the singular measurement of avoidance should not be used, but studies should focus on irritancy, transmission inhibition, antifeedancy and biting dissuasion [2]. Transmission inhibition occurs when a louse comes into contact with, but refuses to transfer onto a treated hair. Antifeedancy describes the behaviour of lice that remain in a treated area of skin but which refuse to imbibe a blood meal even after biting. Biting dissuasion refers to lice that remain on a treated area and which do not attempt to bite.

On the other hand, irritancy manifests in three different ways depending on how an organism responds to a stimulus. These terms are described below [2]:

- Irritant-based *tropotaxis* refers to movement of a louse away from a repellent. Some definitions stipulate that this occurs as a result of comparing sensory input derived from two paired receptors on both sides of the body, however this term is also used in the cellular realm where this does not apply. Negative tropotaxis or movement away from a repellent is classical "avoidance" and is demonstrated when a louse refuses to walk onto a treated portion of hair. When tropotaxis is mild, it manifests as hesitation or reverse in travel by a louse that has already walked onto a treated portion of a hair.

- Irritant-based *orthokinesis* refers to the speed of progress while transversing a treated portion of a hair. It is a response that involves an undirected change in the speed of locomotion of the body as a whole, and/or the frequency of change from rest to movement.

- Irritant-based *klinokinesis* refers to the frequency or amount of changes in the rate of turning from side to side by the whole animal and is indicative of "confusion".

6.10.2. Research on irritant-based tropotaxis

■ Early reports

In the first half of the 20th Century, many studies were conducted with the aim of discovering a repellent for body and head lice [3]. These tests were largely unsuccessful leading researchers to question whether lice possessed the ability to smell. In 1941, however, Wigglesworth employed a methodology that allowed him discern repellent qualities in many experiments using light oils, creosote, naphthalene and shell odourless distillate [3]. He also undertook several studies to determine repellent responses in response to physical stimuli. Head lice were observed to be repelled by temperature lower than 24° C and above 35° C, and relative humidity below 10% and above 75%.

■ Essential oils

Virtually all herbal remedy books and websites providing advice on head lice promote the use of transmission inhibitors that can be applied to the hair to prevent lice infestation. Most pharmacies and alternative health retailers market particular essential oils or blends of these oils from many of these herbs alone and in different combinations. Unfortunately, the repellent effects associated with these oils are only reputed, and very few repellent trials on head lice have been published.

Essential oils from eucalyptus, lavender, rosemary, citronella and some individual components (limonene, geraniol, citronella) were then tested on body lice by Mumcuoglu et al. [4]. They identified citronella as the most promising repellent and tested it in a follow-up study in 2004 on 198 school children in a double-blinded randomised trial during a four-month period [5]. Citronella reduced incidence of infestations from 34-55% down to 12-15% indicating a drop of 66-78%. They concluded that *"an effective repellent could significantly lower the incidence of reinfestations"*. Toloza et al. experimented with a number of derivatives and essential oils from eucalyptus and lavender [6]. The former outperformed the latter by 50% and both were outperformed by piperonal and various aliphatic lactones. There are thousands of species of *Eucalyptus* so results from this oil are of no scientific interest.

■ Phytochemicals

Repellent research employing Wigglesworth's methodology was reinitiated in 1993 by Burgess, Peock and Maunder who experimented with piperonal (heliotropine) on body lice that had been colonised on rabbits for over forty years [7-9]. Piperonal is a common agent in flavours and fragrances, and its pediculicidal properties were first observed in 1918. Burgess claimed that piperonal was 93.3% effective in causing avoidance in body lice, while Peock and Maunder found that piperonal was twice as effective as DEET. These results failed to be replicated in the field in an unpublished, double-blinded, cross-over field trial, involving the participation of over forty families for a six-month period [10]. In addition to essential oils, Mumcouglu et al. also evaluated the repellent efficacy of the individual components, limonene, geraniol and citronella [4]. When tested on body lice, the oil extracted from citronella was observed to exhibit a higher degree of repellent activity.

■ **Aliphatic lactones**

In Toloza et al.'s experiments, three synthetic aliphatic lactones of non-botanical origin were evaluated as head lice repellents *in vitro* and were compared to oils from eucalyptus, lavender and piperonal [6]. Results showed the highest activity for the δ-dodecalactone (repellency index 76.68), which was significantly better from the repellent effect of the essential oils discussed in the previous section (repellency index 32-50), but not better than piperonal.

■ **N,N-Diethyl-*meta*-toluamide (DEET)**

DEET was discovered in 1946 by the US Army who used it to protect their soldiers from vector-borne diseases and arthropod infestations in the field. It is a colourless liquid that has a faint odour and does not dissolve easily in water. DEET remains one of the most effective arthropod repellents for use against mosquitoes, biting flies, fleas, ticks and other biting arthropods. In 1957, DEET became available to the public and has since then been a key ingredient in most off-the-shelf repellents. It features both in skin-applied preparations and in material impregnation at concentrations ranging from 5 to 95%.

While DEET-containing personal repellents are undoubtedly the most recommended general anti-insect products, many people prefer not to use them because of skin sensitivities, odour and perceived toxic effects. A number of manufacturers have developed a wide range of botanical alternatives to meet this demand, but there is very little efficacy data on botanicals because they are exempt from governmental registration requirements. Consumers are, however, the driving force because they want to know how well and for how long these products perform. This demand is resulting in some countries requiring proof of efficacy before the product can be sold in retail outlets. DEET is not effective against head lice [2, 11].

In 1994, Ibarra and Williams asserted that DEET is not a true repellent since it *"apparently masks close range location behaviour"* and does not cause *"orientated movements away from its source"* [12]. While they argued that the use of DEET on head lice constituted a *"misunderstanding of its mode of action"*, the fact remains that avoidance is not the only element of repellence.

6.10.3. Factors affecting efficacy and effectiveness

In most mosquito studies using botanical or phytochemical repellents, the duration of protective effect ranges from 2 to 10 hours. This depends mainly on growing conditions, plant part, plant species, pest species, method of extraction, solvents used to extract oils, and the concentration of applied compound [13]. Environmental factors also play a significant role in determining the duration of protection by a repellent since sunlight acts to breakdown chemicals, wind evaporates volatile oils which are usually the active ingredients, and temperature causes different skin emanations which may dilute or chemically alter repellent composition [13]. Head lice, however, introduce a new variable into this issue and that is human behaviour and body effects. The laboratory and field studies on piperonal illustrate the difficulties inherent in trials with infested human subjects who regularly become re-infested after treatment and whose hair is frequently exposed to wetting and drying agents along with numerous additional chemicals. The survival adaptations of head lice [14] confer a great deal of protection in the field while they are perhaps less effective in the laboratory. There is thus a significant gap between efficacy and effectiveness when it comes to head lice.

6.10.4. Research on other repellent mechanisms

Unfortunately, most head lice researchers have focused on *in vitro* avoidance. An exception to this can be found in a recent study by Canyon et al. [2]. In this study, 150 to 260 adult lice recently harvested from school children and maintained on blood were used in each of three experiments. The repellents tested were:

- Coconut oil (*Cocos nucifera*)
- Coconut oil, neem seed oil (*Azadirachta indica*), citronella oil (*Cymbopogon nardus*)
- Neem seed oil, citronella oil

- Quitnit [tea tree whole plant oil (*Melaleuca alternifolia*), lavender oil (*Lavendula augustifolia*), rosemary oil (*Rosemarinus officinalis*), citronella, neem]
- Scalp Oil [rosemary, bay oil (*Laurus nobilis*), cedarwood oil (*Juniperus virginiana*), patchouli oil (*Pogostemon cablin*), ylangylang oil (*Cananga odorata*), jojoba oil (*Simmondsia chinensis*), apricot oil (*Prunus armeniaca*)]
- Tea Tree oil
- Peppermint oil (*Mentha piperita*)
- Lavender oil
- KY-Jelly (lubricant control)
- DEET 6.6% (Skintastic®)

In the first experiment, the efficacy of a repellent in preventing transmission was assessed by placing lice in the middle of a hair that was coated in repellent on both ends. Another repellent-treated hair was passed by at 4 m/sec laterally, tail-to-head, in contact with lice on the suspended hair (☞ Figure 6.13).

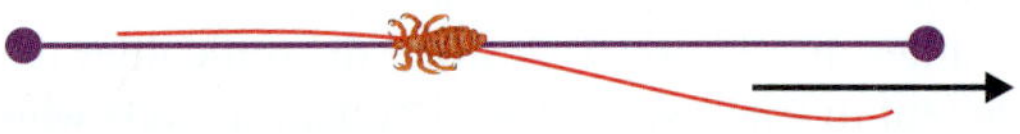

Figure 6.13: Description of experimental procedure in experiment one (1).

Transmission was assessed in terms of successful transfer into passing hair or unsuccessful transfer [1] and results are shown in Table 6.1. In the second experiment, the efficacy of a repellent as an irritant was assessed by placing lice in the middle of a hair that was coated in repellent on both ends (☞ Figure 6.14).

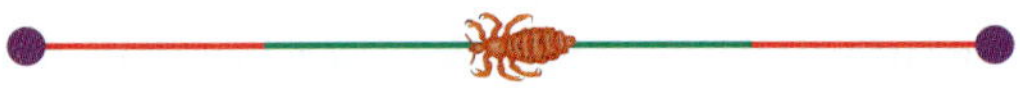

Figure 6.14: Description of experimental procedure in experiment two (2).

The response was assessed as "*normal, very mild, mild, moderate, strong*" increases in tropotaxis (hesitation and avoidance). Response was also assessed in terms of normal, mild or strong: deceases in rate of movement (orthokinesis) and increases in rate of direction change (klinokinesis). In the third experiment, the efficacy of a repellent in preventing bites and blood feeding was assessed by placing lice in the middle of a repellent-treated area (3 cm²) on the author's forearm. *In vitro* arena tests omit the attractive host so their results cannot be extrapolated to reality. Here, repellence was assessed by lice leaving or staying within the treated area of skin and antifeedance was assessed by observing whether or not lice bloodfed in the treated area or remained in the treated area without bloodfeeding. Results are depicted in Table 6.1. This study found that all substances tested were not sufficiently efficacious as head lice repellents with only a marginal level of activity demonstrated (☞ Table 6.6).

Although the tested substances reduced transmission onto a treated hair by 33-65%, most of this effect was due to the slippery nature of treated hair as demonstrated by the KY-Jelly response. The blend of coconut, neem and citronella was most efficacious at preventing transfer while other substances completely failed. As a control, DEET was outperformed in all tests and completely failed as a repellent. Coconut induced the greatest increase in tropotaxis and klinokinesis, however, neem and citronella were less important irritants and reduced the irritancy of coconut when combined. There were no clear winners for orthokinesis with scalp oil performing marginally better due to its extremely viscous nature.

In the repellent skin tests, tea tree and peppermint were superior, however this result may be easily misinterpreted. Once a louse transfers onto a head, it will be repelled by areas of skin that are covered by this repellent and will move to an untreated area or will depart the host. In the antifeedent skin tests, lavender emerged as clearly superior. This means that a louse recently transferred onto a lavender-treated head will not be repelled from treated areas and will not be inclined to feed on them. Since lice are highly mobile, this will eventually result in the lice identifying an untreated area or they will depart the host. Another possibility is that lice will simply go into stasis (physiological shutdown) and will wait for better conditions when the hair is washed [14]. It may well be that other combinations designed to have several repellent effects may prove to be more efficacious.

6.10.5. Area repellents

The above-mentioned repellents are mostly topical lotions and formulations. Area repellents are

6.10. Head lice repellents

Summary of Results Scale (1-10, low to high)	Exp 1 Transfer limited	Exp 2 Irritant	Exp 3 Repellent	Exp 3 Anti-feedant
Coconut, Neem, Citronella	xxxxxxxx	xxxx		
Peppermint	xxxxxxx	x	xxxx	
DEET 6.6% (Skintastic) (+ve control)	xxxxxxx	xxx	xxx	
Quitnit (tea tree, lavender, rosemary, citronella, neem)	xxxxxxx	xxx		
Coconut oil	xxxxxx	xxxxxx	xx	
Scalp Oil (rosemary, bay, cederwood, patchouli, ylang ylang, jojoba, apricot)	xxxxxx	xxxx	xx	
Tea Tree	xxxxx	xx	xxxxx	xx
Lavender	xxxx		x	xxxx
Neem, Citronella	xxxx	xxx		x
KY-Jelly (lubricant control)	xxxxx	x		
Control (no skin treatment)			all stayed	all fed

Table 6.6: Summary of repellent testing results scored out of ten with control effects shown in red. The irritancy score was derived from summing tropotaxis, orthokinesis and klinokinesis.
Prevention of transfer is perhaps the most fundamental of issues when it comes to head lice infestations.

another type and used in two ways with the first being to create an environmental barrier between potential hosts and the arthropods seeking them out. The second method involves the use of evaporative or smoke-based area repellents. These are very common throughout the Australia-Asia-Pacific region for insect control, while they are somewhat overlooked in the USA and Europe. Most contain allethrin and several now incorporate botanical substances with unknown effect.

The use of area repellents is particularly effective against arthropods, such as some species of mosquitoes, which have a tendency to rest on the walls in a house before or after host-seeking and blood-feeding. They also work well on ground-based arthropods, such as ticks and fleas.

Area repellents are frequently overlooked in the arsenal of personal protection measures, but there are several such products on the market accompanied by the expected paucity of comparative and empirical data on their effectiveness.

This type of repellent is mentioned here because of the persistent assertion and/or myth that head lice persist for a short time in the environment and transmit via fomites [1]. On the contrary, if one accepts that the main source of transmission is due to head-to-head contact, the usefulness of area repellents appears negligible.

6.10.6. Lice repellents in humans

When the author began working on head lice in 2002, it became apparent that researchers were entirely dependent on harvesting lice in the field for all experiments and that laboratory-based colonisation was not available. Lice were thus placed on the author's head multiple times in an effort to initiate a colony. These efforts were entirely unsuccessful on this person, but successful on others. Within a week of becoming infested, no nymph or adult stages could be found and only eggs remained. Around this time, a new human-based repellent was inadvertently discovered by US Army mosquito repellent researchers, which prompted the author to consider the possibility that some people are naturally resistant to head lice and exude powerful, effective and natural repellents or pediculicides. Since the author did not repel mosquitoes, this natural was thought to be a different chemical(s) or internal instead of on the skin. Further, it has been observed that 10-15% of all lice feeding on the author and on a colleague experience internal haemorrhaging resulting in subsequent death.

In 2004, the author travelled to Satawal Island in the Federated States of Micronesia for the purpose of collecting mosquitoes during an outbreak of lymphatic filariasis. It was found that most of the four hundred inhabitants were infested with head lice for which social grooming behaviours had been developed. Upon asking if anybody never was infested, an affirmative answer was received. At least ten women were perpetually and completely free of head lice and had to reinfest themselves regularly to take part in the social grooming and bonding practices. Further studies are required to determine if a human-based repellent is the cause of these observations or if there is a degree of "immunity".

6.10.7. Final considerations

Since a single gravid louse is sufficient to initiate an infestation, the requirement for an effective repellent is set very high at close to one hundred percent. Any reduction in transmission, however impressive, will not necessarily protect an individual or prevent infestations in a given population.

It must be stated that any application of repellent or other preventative in infested individuals may act to increase the dispersal of head lice to other contacts in social groups or family. Head lice are thought to view people's heads as "rooms" in their "home" rather than viewing a head as a permanent abode [2]. Core social groups in classrooms probably facilitate this behaviour. Increased dispersal within the core group would thus cause a more rapid change of rooms with greater potential to infest subsidiary contact groups. So, application of preventatives to all subsidiary groups and family would be beneficial only if combined with identification and thorough treatment of all core group members.

There are currently no functional head lice repellents available and all products claiming that they are effective repellents do so facetiously. However, this does not mean that the search for an effective repellent should cease. On the positive side, arthropods have not shown any signs of developing "resistance" to repellents so this is not expected in head lice. The gauntlet has been thrown and future areas for research have been delineated, but head lice researchers are often self funded and so things will progress slowly unless industry assumes a significant role or head lice start vectoring a disease. The challenge is significant because a head lice repellent needs to be close to perfect to be worth using.

6.10.8. References

1. Canyon DV, Speare R, Muller R. Spatial and kinetic factors for the transfer of head lice (*Pediculus capitis*) between hairs. J Invest Dermatol 2002; 119:629-31.

2. Canyon DV, Speare R. A comparison of botanical and synthetic substances commonly used to prevent head lice (*Pediculus humanus* var. *capitis*) infestation. Int J Dermatol 2007;46:422-6.

3. Wigglesworth VB. The sensory physiology of the human louse *Pediculus humanus corporis* De Geer (Anoplura). Parasitol 1941;33:67-109.

4. Mumcuoglu KY, R. Galun, U. Bach, Miller J, Magdassi. S. Repellency of essential oils and their components to the human body louse, *Pediculus humanus humanus* (Anoplura: Pediculidae). Entomol Exp Appl 1996;78: 309-14.

5. Mumcuoglu KY, Magdassi S, Miller J, Ben-Ishai F, Zentner G, Helbin V, et al. Repellency of citronella for head lice: double-blind randomized trial of efficacy and safety. Isr Med Assoc J 2004;6: 756-9.

6. Toloza AC, Zygadlo J, Mougabure-Cueto G, Zerba E, Faillaci S, Picollo MI. The fumigant and repellent activity of aliphatic lactones against *Pediculus humanus capitis* (Anoplura: Pediculidae). Mem Inst Oswaldo Cruz 2006; 101:55-6.

7. Burgess I. New head louse repellent. Br J Dermatol 1993;128:357-60.

8. Burgess I. The function of repellent in head louse control. Pharm J 1993;15:674-5.

9. Peock S, Maunder JW. Arena tests with piperonal, a new louse repellent. J R Soc Promot Health 1993;113: 292-4.

10. Burgess I. Head lice. Clin Evid 2004:2168-73.

11. Rossini C, Castillo L, Gonzalez A. Plant extracts and their components as potential control agents against human head lice. Phytochem Rev 2008;7:51-63.

12. Ibarra J. Coping with head lice in the 1990s. Primary Health Care 1994;4:19-21.

13. Shaalan EA, Canyon D, Younes MW, Abdel-Wahab H, Mansour AH. A review of botanical phytochemicals with mosquitocidal potential. Environ Int 2005;31:1149-66.

14. Canyon DV, Speare R. Do head lice spread in swimming pools? Int J Dermatol 2007; 46:1211-3.

6.11. Potential for future treatments targeting endosymbionts of head lice

Symbiotic relationships are biological interactions between two different organisms in which both organisms benefit. Endosymbiosis describes relationships where organisms, such as bacteria, live inside other organisms. Bacterial symbionts, which not only need their host to survive and prosper but also may be essential to the survival of their hosts, have been cited in the literature for at least 10% of insect species [1]. Symbionts are divided into two categories—primary and secondary. Primary symbionts are essential for host survival while secondary symbionts are not [2].

To better understand the bacterial symbionts of head lice, which have been difficult to culture in the past, researchers have been studying the 16s RNA gene and comparing it to similar bacteria. Through these studies, a dominant primary symbiont (*Candidatus Burkhart pediculicola*) has been found to exist for head lice [1, 3, 4]. A secondary symbiont, *Wolbachia pipientis* has been described previously [5]. A group of cells (organs) of invertebrates that host bacterial or fungal symbionts are called mycetomes. In head lice, the main mycetome is the stomach disc, and the same bacteria in the stomach disc can also be found in the ovaries of female head lice, allowing for vertical transmission of the lice symbiont [1, 6]. During the life cycles of head lice, the primary symbiotic bacteria alternate between intracellular and extracellular spaces, are housed in different mycetomes (including two different transport mycetomes), and at one point, have to outrun the host's immune system [6]. Researchers have demonstrated the migration of symbionts from the stomach disc to the ovarian ampullae, then to the individual oocytes of head lice [3, 6]. Therefore, symbiotic bacteria are present throughout all stages of development of head lice.

Burkhart (2003), Sasaki-Fukatsu (2006) and Perotti (2007) have better described the primary bacterial symbiont of human head lice [1, 3, 6]. This bacterium is a gamma-Proteobacterium [1], belonging to the family Enterobacteriaceae. The same bacterium is also found in body lice. The primary symbiotic bacteria start as rod-shaped organisms, before growing 20 to 50 times their original size to become more filamentous in shape [6]. Proteobacteria are all gram negative bacteria that are facultatively or obligately anaerobic. Some other bacteria within this same group include *Salmonella, E. coli, Yersinia pestis*, and *Pseudomonas*.

Because vertebrate blood lacks certain nutrients such as Vitamin B, symbionts are postulated to help blood-feeding insects obtain these missing nutrients [3]. Symbiotic bacteria help head lice generate thiamine, riboflavin, nicotinic acid, pyridoxine, and pantothenic acid [1]. Although yet to be documented in head lice, symbionts have also been shown to produce proteins and antimicrobial substances that help insects fight off other pathogens and develop resistance to insecticides [7]. Conversely, host insects have been shown to help make or obtain amino acids and minerals which are useful for the bacteria [8].

Survival of head lice, at all points in their life cycles, appears dependent on survival of their primary symbionts. To elucidate the importance of the primary symbiont to head lice, researchers found that male head lice, that are deficient in mycetomes, do not survive more than six days [9]. Dislodged mycetomes, secondary to centrifugation of body louse eggs, lead to the demise of the lice within six days after the eggs have hatched [9].

Considering these facts, it may be possible to eradicate head lice by targeting their bacterial symbionts. Targeting bacterial symbionts in the treatment of head lice could possibly lead to less toxic treatment modalities than standard insecticides, which all have neurotoxicities. In addition, some of the most widely used treatments for head lice, such as permethrin, often have not been efficacious secondary to resistance caused by mutations in the voltage-sensitive sodium channel in the nervous system [10].

Researchers have used antibiotics to target insect endosymbionts throughout nature. For example, studies on *Wigglesworthia glossinidia* (primary endosymbiont that became sterile when treated with ampicillin or tetracycline) and *Sodalis glossinidius* (secondary endosymbiont that had reduced longevity when targeted by streptozotocin), endosymbionts of the tsetse fly, have had promising results [11]. In addition, antibiotic treatment of the aphid host, which eliminates the endosymbiont, reduces aphid growth and induces sterility [12].

Although symbiotic bacteria have lineages similar to categories of free-living bacteria, their deoxyribonucleic acid sequences are distinct from these bacteria. They have evolved into their unique niche as symbionts—some for millions of years—relying on their host for their survival and vice versa [9]. Therefore they have been isolated from the external world for millions of years and do not have the same reaction to antibiotics that other bacteria have had. Antibiotics thus far have not successfully eliminated bacterial symbionts. In addition, insects have shown tolerance to different doses of antibiotics [9]. In short, although larval growth and embryogenesis are slowed *in vivo* in the presence of antibiotics, complete aposymbiosis is not achieved with antibiotics [9].

The most studied antibiotic for head lice treatment is trimethoprim-sulfamethoxazole (co-trimoxazole). Reports have been somewhat dismal in terms of its efficacy. Hipolito et al. (2001) found that for multiple treatment failures, a combination of permethrin 1% cream and oral co-trimoxazole could help eradicate head lice better when compared to either treatment alone [13]. However, Sim et al. (2001) found no difference in the efficacy when treating patients with a combination of lindane and co-trimoxazole, compared to lindane alone [14]. Morsy et al. (1996) attempted to use co-trimoxazole for the treatment of head lice and found that at the end of their seven day treatment period, patients still continued to have head lice infestations. In addition, 3 of 14 patients had dropped out of the study secondary to side effects such as gastrointestinal symptoms [15]. Therefore, not only was co-trimoxazole ineffective in eradicating head lice, it also produced intolerable side effects. Finally, although oral antibiotics may have some effect on adult lice, the nits are still not affected; thus, repeated treatments may be necessary.

Now that more information about endosymbionts of human head lice is available, we can begin to explore other therapeutic choices that target endosymbionts. Some have proposed the alteration of hormones and temperature and the development of a vaccine targeted against symbionts to ultimately eradicate their host. Anti-juvenile hormone KK-4 can decrease female fertility by diminishing the number of eggs and cause absence of chorionation of eggs [9]. Meanwhile, the eggs of some insects cannot adapt to changes in temperature as they cannot aerate their inner organs well. Therefore, high temperature is not well tolerated in symbionts dwelling in eggs as opposed to adult insects. The alteration of temperature could be used in conjunction with other treatments to target both hatched head lice and their eggs. Finally, it may be possible to develop a vaccine against insects via their symbionts. Symbiotic bacteria could be genetically transformed to express molecules with antiparasitic activity before introduction to their insect hosts. Symbiotic bacteria would help transport these lethal genes, leading to the demise of head lice [9]. The role of basic research is pertinent to further understand and develop these treatments. In conclusion, better understanding—and more accurate classification—of primary bacterial symbionts of head lice may lead to the development of more effective eradication methods.

Acknowledgements: Special thanks to Dr. Dean Morrell, Department of Dermatology, University of North Carolina at Chapel Hill, for reviewing this chapter.

6.11.1. References

1. Burkhart, CN. Nit Sheath and Bacterial Symbiotes of *Pediculus humanus capitis* (the Human Head Louse) [master's thesis]. Toledo (OH): Medical College of Ohio; 2003. p. 13-16, 19, 21, 25-27, 29, 58, 63-66.

2. Moran NA and Baumann P. Bacterial endosymbionts in animals. Curr Opin Microbiol 2000,3:270-5.

3. Sasaki-Fukatsu K, Koga R, Nikoh N, Yoshizawa K, Kasai S, Mihara M, Kobayashi M, Tomita T, Fukatsu T. Symbiotic bacteria associated with stomach discs of human lice. Appl Environ Microbiol 2006,72:7349-52.

4. Burkhart CN. Head lice, symbiotic bacteria, the Journal of Cutaneous Medicine and Surgery, and taxonomic precedence. J Cutan Med Surg 2008,12:49.

5. Kyei-Poku GK, Colwell DD, Coghlin P, Benkel B, Floate KD. On the ubiquity and phylogeny of Wolbachia in lice. Mol Ecol 2005,14:285-94.

6. Perotti MA, Allen JM, Reed DL, Braig HR. Host-symbiont interactions of the primary endosymbiont of human head and body lice. FASEB J 2007,21:1058-66.

7. Douglas AE. Mycetocyte symbiosis in insects. Biol Rev Camb Philos Soc 1989,64:409-34.

8. Dadd RH. The nutritional requirements of locusts. III. Carbohydrate requirements and utilization. J Insect Physiol 1960,5:301-16.

9. Burkhart CN, Burkhart CG. Bacterial symbiotes, their presence in head lice, and potential treatment avenues. J Cutan Med Surg 2006,10:2-6.

10. Lee SH, Gao J, Yoon, KS, Mumcuoglu KY, Taplin D, Edman JD, Takano-Lee M, Clark JM. Sodium channel mutations associated with knockdown resistance in the human head louse, *Pediculus capitis* (De Geer). Pest Biochem Physiol 2003,75:79-91.

11. Dale C, Welburn SC. The endosymbionts of tsetse flies: manipulating host-parasite interactions. Int J Parasitol 2001,31:628-31.

12. Houk, EJ and Griffiths, GW Common molecular mechanisms of symbiosis and pathogenesis. Trends Microbiol 1980,8:2226-2231.

13. Hipolito RB, Mallorca FG, Zuniga-Macaraig ZO, Apolinario PC, Wheeler-Sherman. Head lice infestation: single drug versus combination therapy with one percent permethrin and trimethoprim/sulfamethoxazole. J Pediatrics 2001,107:E30.

14. Sim S, Lee IY, Lee KJ, Seo JH, Im KI, Shin MH, Yong TS. A survey on head lice infestation in Korea (2001) and the therapeutic efficacy of oral trimethoprim/sulfamethoxazole adding to lindane shampoo. Korean J Parasitol 2003,41:57-61.

15. Morsy TA, Ramadan NI, Mahmoud MS, Lashen AH. On the efficacy of Co-trimoxazole as an oral treatment for pediculosis capitis infestation. J Egypt Soc Parasitol 1996,26:73-7.

6.12. Is immunisation the future of louse control?

Humans have tried various methods for control of head lice and hitherto most have sequentially failed. It was somewhat inevitable that apart from individual successes, as a result of diligence and vigilance, combing could not be an adequate treatment method for communities irrespective of when it was used in human history. Similarly, physiologically acting insecticides were all doomed to suffer detoxification by the insects and misuse by consumers. Thus the continual competition between insect and insecticide as to whether the insect is killed before it detoxifies the insecticide or the insecticide is metabolised before it kills the insect ultimately swings in favour of the insects. The fact that most people find diagnosis of the infestation at an early stage, before the lice have laid eggs and the numbers increased, extremely difficult, thus allowing the infestation to spread through the community. Therefore a more predictable and reliable method for treating is what most people are seeking.

Ectoparasites by their very nature, with a haematophagous habit that results in exposure of the host to immunogenic salivary proteins and antigenic components of faeces, induce some level of immune response in their host. That immunity affects the interaction between the host and the louse —but to what degree? Could the immune response be used to protect from infestation?

Immunisation against head lice could hypothetically provide the protection from infestation that many parents feel they might want. However, immunisation presents a number of challenges both of a practical scientific and medical nature and of a philosophical and ethical nature. Immunisation of hosts to ectoparasites has been developed to salivary, gut components, and somatic antigens in the field of animal husbandry, such as in control of cattle ticks, but in the main this approach has limitations. Immunisation against both endoparasites and ectoparasites in ruminants is effective for a limited period and generally requires re-immunisation at regular intervals in order to give acceptable protection.

The first point of contact between a louse and its host is via the bite that enables lice to obtain blood. During this process saliva is injected into the host to inhibit haemostasis. Other arthropods use a variety of strategies to facilitate blood feeding including vasodilatation, platelet aggregation inhibition, and suppression of fibrin formation. Each of these strategies may employ various chemical mediators, which have been identified in some species but have not yet been elucidated for human lice. These materials are highly immunogenic and, as well as inhibiting blood clotting, are also responsible for the host immune response that results in the various maculopapular reactions that are related to insect bites. However, it is relatively clear that this form of immunisation has no clinical influence on either survival of lice or of maintenance of an infestation because many people progress through various stages of the development of maculopapular response, even to immune tolerance in some cases, but still suffer an infestation of similar intensity.

Immunisation of rabbits with mid gut extracts has been demonstrated to reduce blood feeding, increase mortality, delay nymphal development, and reduce fecundity of adult body lice but the insects were able to survive [1]. The nine antigens found on microvilli of the gut epithelial cells were found to have four that appeared to be in common from the eight antigens extracted from louse faeces [2-4]. When faecal extracts were used to immunise rabbits, giving a titre of 1:10000, a similar inhibitive effect on development rates of juveniles, fecundity of females, and blood meal ingestion was observed as using mid gut extract [5]. However, in none of these investigations was the acquired immunity sufficient to prevent lice from surviving or from developing from one stage to another. This raises a question as to whether attacking gut antigens is a reasonable approach for preventing or controlling infestations simply because it allows infestation to occur and survive for some time. This might be acceptable for cattle or sheep, in which none of the vaccines developed against ticks or lice completely protects against infestation in much the same way that residual insecticide deposits do not protect completely or consistently and primarily reduce the infestation burden to an acceptable level. But this is not likely to be acceptable in humans who have a "zero tolerance" attitude to infestation.

Of course attempts to immunise hosts against human lice so far have been relatively unsophisticated and have only sought to utilise relatively non-critical antigenic targets by means of humoral responses. It could be possible to target specific cellular receptors or symbiotic microorganisms that would ultimately result in greater disruption of any lice invading the host by means of cytotoxic killer cells. However, there are likely to be important limitations whatever pathway is employed.

Immunisation against microorganisms is well established and from that experience it is clear that in general terms anti-viral immunisation is more long lasting than anti-bacterial immunisation. Also immunisation directed against cellular organisms like bacteria often develops a more limited protection, sometimes with somewhat unpredictable outcomes, for example anti-cholera vaccine is of such limited activity that it is now mostly only used during disease outbreaks as a "fire-break" measure in attempts to limit transmission. Therefore, irrespective of how effective an anti-louse vaccine could be it is likely it would require frequent booster doses in order to maintain acceptable efficacy.

The other main limitation is likely to be related to non-specific action, possibly triggered by other biting insects that utilise similar salivary proteins or have similar somatic antigens. Any kind of anamnestic immune response that is triggered only irregularly, if at all, may be not only slow to activate but also unpredictable in outcome or potency. Insect bite reactions may trigger such unpredictable events. For example, the commonly encountered delayed hypersensitivity reaction resulting in a maculopapular reaction may also have a cytotoxic component resulting in a vesicular or bullous response. Such a response appears to have little effect on lice. Young nymphs that are not disturbed, particularly those of the crab louse *Pthirus pubis*, often remain in one place for several days at a time, triggering pronounced bullous responses that may almost envelope the insect yet they remain viable and continue to feed, apparently at the normal rate (I.F. Burgess, unpublished). Consequently, it is likely that cytotoxic reactions developed against lice may have the unfortunate consequence of accidentally increasing host pathology through non-specific side effects.

Ultimately it is the philosophical and ethical factors that will decide whether immunisation against lice is a reasonable proposition. Interesting as it may be from a scientific point of view, and however positive may be researchers that they can develop an effective and efficient vaccine, the final decision in this will be the parents of the children at risk. Irrespective of any other factors such as annoyance, social stigma, and the minor pathology arising from continuous biting, head louse infestation is not a life threatening condition. Even the dubious possibility that under the right circumstances the insects could be the vectors of disease does not make them important pathogens. Balance this against the possible negative aspects of immunisation and it becomes increasingly difficult to define an argument that can honestly support developing an anti-head louse vaccine. In some countries there is already increasing disaffection with immunisation against considerably more serious infections such as measles, mumps, and rubella amongst parents and carers. As a result numbers of measles cases are currently higher than they have been for more than a decade. Therefore, to add, even as an option, a further vaccine to an already crowded schedule of immunisations may just be one step too far for some people or communities. Add to this the relatively high probability that however effective the vaccine is that it will not actually prevent infestation from occurring, even if it prevents that infestation from developing fully. Such an activity may ultimately reduce or even eliminate transmission in a community but in order to do so would require a high proportion of families in the community to participate, and in most countries this is just not likely to happen, so the future of louse control doubtless lies elsewhere.

6.12.1. References

1. Ben-Yakir D, Mumcuoglu KY, Manor O, Ochanda JO, Galun R. Immunization of rabbits with a midgut extract of the human body louse *Pediculus humanus humanus*: the effect of induced resistance on the louse population. Med Vet Entomol 1994;8:114-118.

2. Ochanda JO, Mumcuoglu KY, Ben-Yakir D, Okuru JK, Oduol VO, Galun R. Characterization and properties of body louse midgut antigenic proteins recognized by resistant hosts. Med Vet Entomol 1996;10:35-38.

3. Mumcuoglu KY, Ben-Yakir D, Gunzberg S, Ocbanda JO, Galun R. Immunogenic proteins in the body and faecal material of the human body louse, *Pediculus humanus*, and their homology to antigens of other lice species. Med Vet Entomol 1996;10:105-107.

4. Mumcuoglu KY, Rahamim E, Ben-Yakir D, Ochanda JO, Galun, R. Localization of immunogenic antigens on midgut of the human body louse *Pediculus humanus humanus* (Anoplura: Pediculidae). J Med Entomol 1996; 33:74-77.

5. Mumcuoglu KY, Ben-Yakir D, Ochanda JO, Miller J, Galun R. Immunization of rabbits with faecal extract of *Pediculus humanus*, the human body louse: effects on louse development and reproduction. Med Vet Entomol 1997;11:315-318

6.13. General considerations on treatments and treatment schemes

Evidence-based treatment of head lice infestations needs to take into consideration the parasite's life cycle. Head lice eggs take 7-12 days to hatch, and the period from first instar larva to egg-laying adult is about 9-11 days [1]. If a pediculicide does not kill embryos in eggs, treatment needs to be repeated after lice have hatched (i.e., after seven or more days), but before the earliest hatched lice have become mature, mated and started to produce eggs (i.e., about 10 days). Thus, there is a narrow window of treatment opportunity (day 7 to 10) for retreatment, assuming no reinfestation.

Most manufacturers recommend retreatment at day 7. A week makes biological sense, and consumers find it easier to remember. It may, however, mean that lice may emerge after the second treatment, if they were 1 or 2 days old when the first treatment was given and were slower to hatch [2]. A single application is only recommended if the product kills all embryos in eggs.

Biology of head lice, however, is only one factor that determines how pediculosis is treated. By far the major determinant is social, particularly the societal attitude towards head lice and within that society, the individual's attitude. In many developing countries, for example, head lice are not regarded adversely and offer positive opportunities for mutual grooming. In some minority populations in developed countries, such as traditional Australian Aboriginal communities, head lice can be a good social lubricant [3]. In developed market economies parents and guardians find the amount of time required to treat head lice frustrating [4]. For details on these aspects see Chapters 9.1. and 9.2. on control of pediculosis and Chapter 7. on sociocultural dimensions.

We would expect that an ideal head lice treatment product would have the following essential and desirable characteristics.

▶ Essential characteristics

- 100% efficacy in killing nymphs and adult lice
- 100% efficacy in killing embryos in eggs
- Good safety and adverse effects profile
- Easy to administer or apply
- High acceptability to users, both person applying and person receiving (e.g., parent and child)
- Good environmental profile (since treatments typically enter the waste water system)
- Low cost
- Low likelihood of current resistance

▶ Desirable characteristics

- Single treatment or application
- Removes eggs
- Requires minimal time to use (<5 min)
- Prevents reinfestation by repelling, not killing, lice
- Low risk of resistance developing

- Appropriate for simultaneous group treatment

Some new treatments meet the essential criteria, but no current treatments meet all essential and desirable criteria. Many topical treatments use a methodology based in antiquity: nit combs and presumably application of liquids to hair have been used to control pediculosis for over 2000 years [5]. In general, topical treatments for head lice have focused on achieving high adulticidal and ovicidal effect. Adulticidal efficacy has been achieved with many neurotoxic, physical and natural products, but ovicidal efficacy of most products is low or has not been tested systematically. The new compounds that meet the essential criteria are dimeticone and spinosad (☞ Table 6.7), but only dimeticone is commercially available. Ivermectin does not kill eggs when used orally, but meets the other essential and several desirable criteria, except in some developed market economies where it is expensive owing to a monopoly situation. Other compounds, such as pyrethroids, pyrethrum, malathion and carbaryl, will probably lose their importance, mainly due to emerging insecticide resistance, perceived toxicity of chemical insecticides, negative impact on the environment and/or the availability of products that meet more of the essential criteria.

Some insecticides are not acceptable at all. The organochlorine insecticide lindane should not be used in humans due to its unacceptable potential to cause toxic effects. In addition, resistance of head lice to lindane increased rapidly over the last years of its availability [6]. Many countries have banned the medical use of lindane and abandoned its use in agriculture owing to its long half-life. As a consequence, lindane-based compounds have been consistently withdrawn from the markets. In Brazil, the use of lindane in agriculture was prohibited in 1985, and on humans in 1998. As late as in 2006, the US-American Environmental Protection Agency (EPA) called for the voluntary cancellation of all agricultural uses of lindane due to its toxic effect on humans and the environment. The European Union prohibited the use of lindane as a pediculicide only by the end of 2007.

In Table 6.7, we have used a semi-quantitative scoring system to grade head lice treatments against the essential and desirable criteria. We think scoring head lice treatments using criteria other than just efficacy at killing lice reflects more accurately how people utilise head lice products since it takes into account a range of factors that individuals consider when choosing a treatment [4]. Most attributes are rated as 3 with a grading of zero if attribute is not met at all, 1 if it is met to some extent, 2 for a moderate extent and 3 for completely met. However, killing of lice and eggs are weighted most heavily (10 rather than 3) since these are the most important criteria under a biological model of pediculosis control. Some newer treatments have not yet been commercialised widely (dimeticone) or at all (spinosad, topical ivermectin), while others require a doctors' prescription in some countries (carbaryl, oral ivermectin, trimethoprim-sulphamethoxazole). Oral treatments score highly on ease of administration, while any treatment that involves careful application of a product to hair with duration of treatment greater than 5 minutes did not score highly. Since cost depends on the marketing structure within a country and is relative to income, we gave most commercially available products a score of 2 for low cost and ivermectin and not yet commercialised products a score of 1 (however, ivermectin is very cheap in some countries where multiple brands are available). In this analysis the herbal products, a large and diverse group, have been scored as a group to represent an average. However, some products are more effective than others [2], and the scores may be an underestimate for some and an overestimate for others.

The products that scored best using this system were dimeticone, particularly high concentration products, malathion, ivermectin and spinosad. Dimeticone has been marketed recently in an increasing number of countries. High concentration dimeticone kills lice and also embryos in eggs and thus a single application can be considered as sufficient [7, 8]. Oral ivermectin by its mode of action (ingested with blood meal) can only kill lice and cannot kill embryos in eggs [9]. Hence, a second dose to kill newly hatched lice is needed. Besides easy administration, it has an additional benefit of killing other parasites, such as intestinal helminths and scabies mites, and thus can be very effectively used in mass treatment programs in communities where these problems are endemic [10]. Topical therapy with ivermectin is also effective, and it may be ovicidal, working through direct contact with

6.13. General considerations on treatments and treatment schemes

Criteria	Wet combing	Pyre-throids	Pyre-thrins	Mala-thion	Herbal	Dimeticone high conc	Dimeticone low conc	Ivermectin oral	Ivermectin topical	Spino-sad	Carba-ryl	Oral TS
Essential												
100% kill lice	5	10	10	10	5	10	8	10	10	10	10	4
100% kill eggs	2	2	2	9	5	10	0	0	5	10	0	0
Low likelihood of resistance	3	0	0	1	3	3	3	3	3	3	1	3
Safe	3	2	2	2	2	3	3	3	3	3	1	1
Easy to administer	0	1	1	1	1	2	2	3	1	1	1	3
Acceptability	3	3	3	2	3	3	3	3	3	3	3	3
Good environmental profile	3	2	2	2	3	3	3	3	3	3	2	3
Low cost	3	2	2	2	2	2	2	1*	1*	1	1	2
Easy to access	3	3	3	2	3	2**	2**	2**	0	0	1	1
Total Essential Score	25	25	25	31	27	38	26	27	29	34	20	20
% Essential Score	61.0%	61.0%	61.0%	75.6%	65.9%	92.7%	63.4%	65.9%	70.7%	82.9%	48.8%	48.8%
Desirable												
Single treatment	0	0	0	2	1	3	0	0	1	3	0	0
Removes eggs	2	0	0	0	0	0	0	0	0	0	0	0
Low risk of resistance developing	3	0	0	0	1	3	3	1	1	2	0	0
Requires minimal time	0	1	1	1	1	1	1	3	1	1	1	3
Prevents reinfestation	0	0	0	0	1	0	0	0	0	0	0	0
Appropriate for group treatment	1	2	2	2	2	2	2	3	2	2	0	0
Total Desirable Score	6	3	3	5	6	9	6	7	5	8	1	3
% Desirable Score	33.3%	16.7%	16.7%	27.8%	33.3%	50.0%	33.3%	38.9%	27.8%	44.4%	5.6%	16.7%
Total Ideal Treatment Score	31	28	28	36	33	47	32	34	34	42	21	23
% Ideal	52.5%	47.5%	47.5%	61.0%	55.9%	79.7%	54.2%	57.6%	57.6%	71.2%	35.6%	39.0%

Table 6.7: Semiquantitative scoring of head lice treatments for essential and desirable criteria.
Killing of lice and their eggs = 10 each or proportionally; other criteria scored out of 3; none = 0, some = 1, medium = 2, complete = 3.
Note: Caution should be given in the case of pyrethroids, pyrethrins and malathion, as scoring of killing lice and eggs refers to settings where no resistance occurs. TS = trimethoprim/sulphamethoxazole. (*: only in high income countries, ivermectin is of low cost, score = 3; **: marketed in a limited number of countries).

lice [11, 12]. However, ivermectin is not registered in most countries for treatment of pediculosis. Malathion scored high due to its adulticidal and ovicidal action in settings where resistance does not occur, but as risk of development of resistance is high, it should be used with caution. Spinosad seems to be an effective and safe alternative, but the product has not yet been commercialised for human use.

The results (☞ Table 6.7, Figure 6.15) highlight that no product meets fully all essential criteria for an ideal head lice treatment and that even fewer products meet desirable criteria. Perhaps the ideal treatment cannot be found in a single product. The two most difficult desirable criteria are removal of eggs and repellence. The only technique that removes eggs is combing using specialised combs and lubricating liquid that slides eggs up the hair shaft [13], but achieving 100% clearance is difficult and time consuming. No chemical method for removing eggs has been discovered [14]. Many compounds show a repellent action *in vitro* [15], and one trial has shown efficacy [16], but the practical benefit and applicability of repellents are still a matter of debate (☞ Chapter 6.10.).

6.13.1. References

1. Lebwohl M, Clark L, Levitt J. Therapy for head lice based on life cycle, resistance, and safety considerations. Pediatrics 2007;119:965-974.

2. Heukelbach J, Speare R, Canyon D. Natural products and their application to the control of head lice: an evidence-based review. In: Brahmachari G, editor. Chemistry of natural products: recent trends & developments. First ed. Kerala, India: Research Signpost; 2006. p. 277-302.

3. Trigger DS. Blackfellows, whitefellows and head lice. Newsletter of the Australian Institute of Aboriginal Studies. 1981;15:63-72.

4. Parison JC, Speare R, Canyon D. Uncovering family experiences with head lice: the difficulties of eradication. Open Dermatol J 2008;2:9-17.

5. Mumcuoglu YK, Zias J. Head lice, *Pediculus humanus capitis* (Anoplura: Pediculidae) from hair combs excavated in Israel and dated from the first century B.C. to the eighth century A.D. J Med Entomol 1988;25:545-547.

6. Meinking TL, Taplin D. Infestations: pediculosis. Curr Probl Dermatol 1996;24:157-163.

7. Heukelbach J, Sonnberg S, Mello I, Speare R, Oliveira FA. High ovicidal efficacy of dimeticone pediculicide: new era of head lice treatment. Submitted. 2009.

8. Oliveira FA, Speare R, Heukelbach J. High *in vitro* efficacy of Nyda® L, a pediculicide containing dimeticone. J Eur Acad Dermatol Venereol 2007;21:1325-1329.

9. Glaziou P, Nguyen LN, Moulia-Pelat JP, Cartel JL, Martin PM. Efficacy of ivermectin for the treatment of head lice (Pediculosis capitis). Trop Med Parasitol 1994; 45:253-254.

10. Heukelbach J, Winter B, Wilcke T, Muehlen M, Albrecht S, Oliveira FA, et al. Selective mass treatment with ivermectin to control intestinal helminthiases and

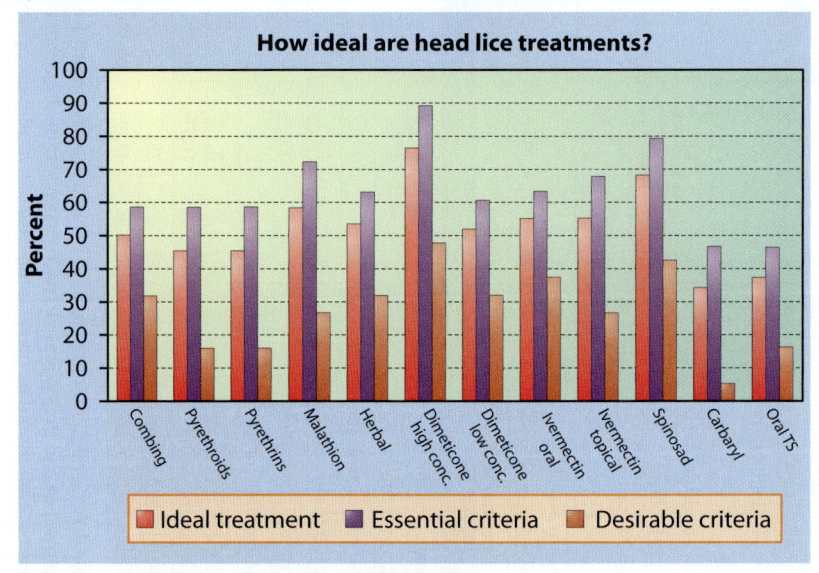

Figure 6.15: Relative essential, desirable and complete score.

parasitic skin diseases in a severely affected population. Bull World Health Organ 2004;82:563-571.

11. Youssef MY, Sadaka HA, Eissa MM, el-Ariny AF. Topical application of ivermectin for human ectoparasites. Am J Trop Med Hyg 1995;53:652-653.

12. Strycharz JP, Yoon KS, Clark JM. A new ivermectin formulation topically kills permethrin-resistant human head lice (Anoplura: Pediculidae). J Med Entomol 2008; 45:75-81.

13. Speare R, Canyon DV, Cahill C, Thomas G. Comparative efficacy of two nit combs in removing head lice (*Pediculus humanus* var. *capitis*) and their eggs. Int J Dermatol 2007;46:1275-1278.

14. Burkhart CN, Burkhart CG. Head lice: scientific assessment of the nit sheath with clinical ramifications and therapeutic options. J Am Acad Dermatol 2005;53:129-133.

15. Canyon DV, Speare R. A comparison of botanical and synthetic substances commonly used to prevent head lice *(Pediculus humanus* var. *capitis)* infestation. Int J Dermatol 2007;46:422-426.

16. Mumcuoglu KY, Magdassi S, Miller J, Ben-Ishai F, Zentner G, Helbin V, et al. Repellency of citronella for head lice: double-blind randomized trial of efficacy and safety. Isr Med Assoc J 2004;6:756-759.

Head Lice and the Impact of Knowledge, Attitudes and Practices—a Social Science Overview

7. Head Lice and the Impact of Knowledge, Attitudes and Practices—a Social Science Overview

The social science investigation of head lice infestations is extremely limited. The neglect of this area of research is mainly due to the fact that this organism has not caused mortality or any significant morbidity in developed societies in contemporary history [1]. From a biomedical point of view it is therefore not a high priority health issue but more a nuisance infection. Research on *Pediculus capitis* focuses overwhelmingly on insect biology, ecology, epidemiology and treatment rather than the sociological impact [2]. Publications for various interest groups create a short list of social science research around this insect for physicians, parents, teachers, school nurses [2].

This chapter presents published and unpublished information from an internet survey conducted by the authors and provides an overview of research on knowledge, attitudes and practices of those who encounter head lice and considers questions yet to be answered.

7.1. Knowledge

Generally, affected people have limited accurate knowledge about head lice and in particular how to treat them. This is clear from a study on 1338 parents in the Australian states of Queensland and Victoria. Only 7% of respondents answered all ten true or false knowledge-based questions correctly, and 64% answered half correctly [3]. Myths were pervasive in this study population. For instance, 70-85% of respondents believed people with head lice scratch their head frequently. Other myths evident were: head lice can jump, are able to survive away from a head for several days, can live in hats or carpet, are selective about their hosts, spread from domestic pets or birds, and the home should be thoroughly cleaned if head lice are found. Just two true treatment-related statements ("treatment needs to involve 2 applications 7 days apart" and "head lice crawl from head to head") were accurately known by a majority of respondents.

In a Brazilian study [4] and the above-mentioned Australian study [3], respondents thought itching was the main symptom that indicated the presence of head lice. The former study asked, *"Do lice transmit disease?"* and 60% of respondents said *"Yes"*.

A variable lack of knowledge was evident in an internet study conducted by the authors in which website visitors were asked a number of questions. In response to the first question, *"What did you hope to find at this website?"*, the major categories of information were: treatment (99.5%), insect biology (38%) and prevention information (8%). While participants were assumed to be lacking in knowledge, since they were searching the internet for more, the range of respondents included the inexperienced to those wanting to locate up-to-date information on treatment. The broad scope of this knowledge search was driven by a desire for effective eradication. Resistance, re-infestation and treatment complexity were the intermediate factors that made this difficult for respondents compelling them to seek more information (see section on practices later in this chapter).

Questions from many respondents revealed the unfortunate widespread dissemination of incorrect information. Individuals searching the web for information are highly conscious of the need for quality and reliability. While the internet contains an encyclopedic volume of information on head lice, most of it is non-authoritative and full of inaccuracies and errors. Notably, a great number of knowledge-based institutions and healthcare organisations derive the information on their websites from non-original sources without discretion or appropriate consideration. For instance, advice to clean fomites upon discovering an infested head is not supported by the evidence-base [5].

7.2. Social attitudes about the infestation

There is a persistent stigma about being infested with head lice that is well accepted anecdotally, but there is little systematic research into this. Stigma is defined by as, *"The degree to which an identity is spoiled as a result of having an illness"* [6]. Psychological literature describes several forms of stigma including: felt stigma, courtesy stigma and enacted stigma [7-10]. Felt stigma is *"when individuals …*

7.2. Social attitudes about the infestation

perceive that they are labeled, stereotyped, and separated from others ..." [10]. Courtesy stigma is stigma by association for family members or close intimates of the individual who bears the stigmatised status. Enacted stigma is experiencing status loss or discrimination as the bearer of a stigmatised status through social policy for example.

Our study sought to gauge the immediate emotional impact. We asked *"what were your feelings upon discovery of head lice?"* [11]. Only a few individuals had a neutral response to the question while the majority had strong negative reactions. Many respondents identified several emotions. The results reflect the variety of emotions expressed by the number of individuals expressing them. It is possible that the replies from a large group of these represent a stigma effect (320 emotional reactions from 294 individuals; ☞ Table 7.1).

Feelings (294 individuals)	n	%
Disgust	64	21.8
Horror	35	11.9
Feel dirty	26	8.8
Frustrated	24	8.2
Anxiety	24	8.2
Anger	14	4.8
Embarrassment	14	4.8
Fear	12	4.1
Very upset	10	3.4
Guilt	10	3.4
Shock	10	3.4
Disappointment	10	3.4
Very annoyed	9	3.0
Shame	7	2.4
Exasperated	6	2.0
Dismay	5	1.7
Other	40	12.2

Table 7.1: Stated feelings on discovery of head lice—strong negative reactions.

The category of "Other" strong feelings (noted in table 1) were: desperate (n=4), urgency to act (n=4), other hygiene perceptions (n=4), hate, overwhelmed, helpless, sick and panic (all n=3), depressed and unhappy (both n=2). Registering one (n=1) mention each were: terrified, appalled, stress, discouraged, *"pissed off"*, disbelief, paranoid, despair, and *"not something people like us get"*.

Feelings that indicated a concern about their identity being spoiled were horror, feel dirty, embarrassed, fear and guilt, shock, panic, shame and dismay. Emotional reactions indicating courtesy stigma were stress, despair, paranoia, fear, shame, feeling overwhelmed, anxiety, anger, embarrassment, dismay, depressed, disappointment and unhappy. Mediocre and neutral reactions were much less common (19% and 10%, respectively).

Respondents feared the exposure and the judgement of others. They were very worried about being labelled or stereotyped and some female parents felt responsible or even guilty for their child. This strong concern compelled some to conceal the infestation for the child's sake. Some parents adopted what they thought was a responsible approach and notified contacts about the infestation. But concern for a stigma based reaction was evident. *"Telling others outside the family who she may have contact with is very awkward"*. Another writer stated she felt *"scared, we have to tell her friends and people assume that you are dirty or low income, which is not the case"*. Others worried that their children might be teased or bullied.

Attitudes about head lice are culturally constructed. These reactions go beyond what is appropriate for such a benign disease. Instead, we see in these emotions about head lice, evidence of socially constructed ideas about cleanliness, disease, public health, parental roles and class-based stereotypes. All these issues are informed by conceptions of the role of the "good citizen" in society which is argued to be central to the maintenance of social order [12]. Talcott Parsons, the North American sociologist, theorised about the ordered society and the importance of value consensus among society members:

"If members of society are committed to the same values, they will tend to share a common identity, which provides a basis for unity and cooperation, and common goals. Values provide a general conception of what is desirable and worthwhile. Goals provide direction in specific situations." [12]

In our study, the respondents demonstrated a value judgement of the undesirability of head lice and their goals for seeking eradication and a return to a parasite-free "normal" health status. Individuals are socialised about the values of society from birth (family, school, work and mass media communications are imbedded with values). Societal roles integrate these values, in particular here the role of the parent. Social equilibrium occurs when people work to affirm and behave according to social values [12]. The stress and action we see evident here with study respondents is the reaction to finding themselves in a negatively viewed social status. In the next section on practice, it is shown that parents act to manage head lice infestations partly to fulfill the role of the good parent by not supporting the spread. Goffman has shown in his research with individuals who have a spoiled identity, whether disclosed or not, that if possible, individuals work to return that identity to "normal" so they fit with the role expectation and a presentation of themselves that is socially acceptable [13]. It is the values and social role expectations embedded in our society that create conditions for stigmatising pediculosis.

Where do these conceptions about lice come from? We must acknowledge the historical antecedents that contribute to stigmatised thinking about lice. In the annals of history lice are linked to rats and plague [1, 14]. We hypothesise that typhus epidemics, crowded living conditions and rat fleas as a vector all figure in the lay public's perception of lice, head or body lice (which we think are confused as one and the same in the public imagination), as something more than a pest. Because of this lice may be perceived as an infestation that can be life threatening to the extent that disease spread by them can decimate populations. The notion of plague is perhaps until recent times the most horrific catastrophe, apart from war, that could be visited upon human populations. Historical analysis has shown that between the European Middle Ages and World War I typhus carried by body lice killed more military combatants than war itself [1]. If this series of propositions are sound then we may have discovered the basis for the strong negative reaction in the general public toward lice.

Mary Douglas' anthropological work which examined cross-culturally the social values around dirt and cleanliness corroborates the social order interpretation [15]. Some traditional societies use classifications of dirt and polluting substances as a means to influence social behaviour, contribute to social order as a social control mechanism, and attribute social status according to bodily pollution status. The Indian caste system is perhaps the most well known example of this. In European and other developed economies the effect of the public health movements would be contributing to social values that compel us to classify lice as a social pollution and undesirable "matter out of place" [15].

Head lice have been used to support other positive social functions. Trigger [16] describes the social bonding role that the head lice grooming ritual constitutes among an Indigenous north Australian social group. Social relationship protocols govern this practice, but it has a very positive role in bonding community members and providing a legitimate excuse for intimacy between family members and other kin or social relationships. Likewise, one of the authors (Canyon) has observed that head lice play an important bonding role in parts of Micronesia and Arnhem Land, Australia where social grooming is commonplace. In Brazilian indigenous populations people often groom each other which strengthens social bonds (J. Heukelbach, personal communication).

Maunder (1987), drawing on psychological literature, makes an interesting case for the influence of human emotional reactions upon the effective eradication of head lice within the human population [17]. Apart from occasional cases of entomophobia, which may also play a role in the reaction, he saw the psychological reaction of *"those who know they have head lice ... and ... those who believe they are free from head lice"* as the main barrier to eradication of the insect. For both groups, he argued that the *"fight/flight reaction"* occurs. For those who know they have a case of head lice, the fight element translates as action to seek to effectively eradicate the insect. Data from our study supports this since treatment with pharmaceutical products was the usual action. The flight element Maunder associates with *"a need for secrecy. Overtones of social shame and the infringement of mores [which] increase the urge to hide the problem from public gaze"* [17]. Maunder sees this as one of the reactions that works to the advantage of the survival of the pest. Concealing head lice infection enables the insect to spread to other hosts and many months can pass before the insect is evident to the new hosts. *"The silence of the donor ensures full use *of that time, by lice, in seeking yet more pastures new".*

In our study, the fight effect for those who think they are free from infection is the unwarranted use of insecticide shampoo and ineffective repellents as prevention measures. Many teachers, child care workers, caring professions and households are afflicted by this reaction. The flight reaction compels a social, emotional and physical distancing between themselves and the potentially infected. Maunder sees this reaction as a basis for a stigma label for those with the infection:

"Therein lies the power house for the creation and perpetuation of the mythology. If dirt, poor personal, hygiene, low class, dubious morals, needing punishment from on High etc., can be linked to having lice. Then all social, emotion and physical distance creation can be made rational and socially acceptable" [17].

The origin of the stigmatised reaction therefore can be understood as a set of complex social processes aimed at creating a social order that protects society from threatening infection. Furthermore, this may be informed by conceptualisations of lice that relate them to plague however incorrect this is in biological reality. The unfortunate effects of action are the marginalisation (self-imposed or by institutions such as schools) or misguided efforts of individuals that are overreactions aimed at achieving eradication.

7.3. Practices

The majority of our study population had some difficulty eradicating the insect. Most study participants sought an immediate solution which they could act upon. There were three categories of issues that affected their ability to achieve their aim of effective eradication. These were technological, biological and social issues (☞ Figure 7.1). However, the population we were able to access through our study were those searching for information. They may have been very new to treating the infection or encountering difficulties or seeking to improve their treatment practice in some way with current information. We did not capture the experience of those who had no difficulty treating head lice [2].

The people who responded to the survey were mainly parents, a few grandparents, guardians and infected or concerned others. They saw the cause of the infection being their child's presence in institutions such as school, day care centre, as well as, the family home among siblings, a perception also evident in the Brazilian study [4].

Technically, the difficulty was finding an effective treatment, concerns about the toxicity of the product with repeated use and the difficulty of treatment methods, particularly with thick, long or curly hair. In the Brazilian study, the problem of selecting an effective treatment was evident in the range of treatments: vinegar, medication, soap,

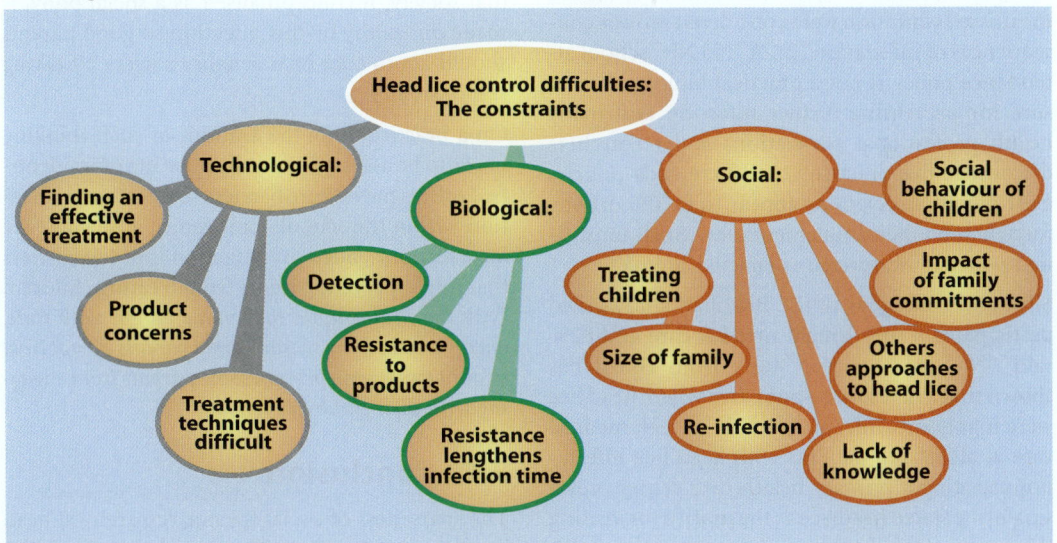

Figure 7.1: Head lice management difficulties [2].

inflammables, oil, herbs, insecticide, and cola soda drink. Physical methods included shaving, manual removal and combing. These respondents used predominantly these physical methods on very young children. The higher income group used vinegar more often and the lower income group used herbs more frequently. Lice combs were used by 85% of respondents and 45% felt able to treat the infection [4].

In our study, the biological challenges were detecting the insect, resistance to pediculicides and prolonged infection time due to resistance and re-infestation. Social barriers to effective eradication were:

- the difficulty of treating young children
- larger sized families translated to a greater treatment workload
- re-infestation compounded the treatment workload
- a lack of knowledge personally and among others
- the social behaviour of children supported ongoing re-infestation
- family commitments where work limited available treatment time
- concern that other parents were not treating their children. There was annoyance and anger expressed about these "others" who do not treat.

Exclusion from school for a quarantine period and the missed education were considered serious consequences of infestation [2]. A "No Nit" school attendance policy is not a practical biological measure for preventing further infection and many health professional associations and researchers discourage this practice [2]. Where such policies exist parent associations appear to be the driving force behind their implementation. Such unjustified policy is interpreted as enacted stigma.

Silva and colleagues in the Brazilian study asked participants if they sought medical care and 82% said "No" [4]. Another study from Brazil has shown that in a resource-poor area where head lice were highly endemic, people did not seek medical care at all: of 110 patients with head lice infestations visiting a primary health care center, not a single one stated head lice as the motive for visiting this service [18]. In this study, in a resource-rich setting, respondents did not mention taking their infection to a doctor either. Approaching pharmacists was the only medically-oriented service identified. Further research needs to confirm the reason carers do not do this. Rationales considered should include: privacy, stigma prevention strategy, thinking it's too trivial for a medical appointment or that doctors consider the infection trivial.

While expenses of commercial treatments for families would be compounded by family size, length of infection period and the type of treatments used, cost was not a major concern in our study on a population drawn from mainly English speaking market economies. Families in lower socio-economic groups might find this more of a burden. Fortunately, treatment options include inexpensive solutions such as generic brand conditioner and a lice comb.

Treating head lice can be seen sociologically as part of the hidden health care system that is the health maintenance conducted in the privacy of the home by in the main female parents [19]. Values about head lice are affirmed and taught to children in the home; this may take the form of social responsibility by notifying others of infestation who may be at risk of transmission or by maintaining a culture of silence to prevent stigma. Values about ethical parenting are also passed on through discussion about the "others" who do not treat and are preventing a normal bodily health status. In essence, this value judgement can be reduced to the idea that society, if conceptualised as a social body, is made unhealthy by this infection so good parents should act to cure or normalise society by taking responsibility.

On a practical level the amount of such thinking needs to be assessed since the blaming of unidentified others may create barriers to effective eradication within the school community. Elsewhere we have recommended investigation into the barriers that might prevent parents from treating children. *"Are the strains upon the female parent with time, energy and cost the reasons some parents do not treat at all? Does stigma prevent some parents from engaging with their children's school?"* [2].

7.4. Conclusion

The sparseness of social science research on head lice is clear and evident. The complexity of treating head lice matches the complexity of social factors that impinge on successful treatment. Most of those involved in the care of head lice cases wish to eradicate head lice completely. However, cultural ideals, social roles, knowledge and practical activities do not always help in achieving this goal. Knowledge and attitudes strongly influence the approach to eradication success or otherwise. The internet can function as the first source of information, but it can be an unreliable one for knowledge seekers. Codes of practice for quality health care information on the internet need to be pursued.

The head louse may be regarded a nuisance by the medical community, but for the lay population it is a complex treatment problem overlaid with a social pariah status that does not assist in the overall eradication of the insect within the human population. As Maunder argued, it is the silence caused by stigma that supports the perpetuation of the species [17].

7.5. References

1. Barnes E. Diseases and Human Evolution. Albuquerque: University of New Mexico Press; 2005.

2. Parison J, Speare R, Canyon DV. Uncovering family experiences with head lice: the difficulties of eradication. The Open Dermatology Journal 2008;2:9-17.

3. Counahan ML, Andrews RM, Weld H, Walsh H, Speare R. What do parents know and do about head lice. Rural and Remote Health [serial on the Internet]. 2007 [cited 2009 Sep 24];7:687+ [about 10 pages]. Available from: http://www.rrh.org.au

4. Silva L, Alencar RA, Madeira NG. Survey assessment of parental perceptions regarding head lice. Int J Dermatol 2008;47:249-255.

5. Speare R, Thomas G, Cahill C. Head lice in pupils of a primary school in Australia and implications for control. Aust N Z J Public Health 2002;26:308-211.

6. Green G, Platt S. (1997). Fear and loathing in health care settings reported by people with HIV. Sociol Health Illn 1997;19:70-92.

7. Miller CT, Kaiser CR. A Theoretical Perspective on Coping with Stigma. J Soc Issues 2001;57:73-92.

8. Scambler G. Sociology, social structure and health-related stigma. PPsychol Health Med 2006; 11:288-295.

9. Herek GM. Thinking about AIDS and Stigma: A Psychologists's Perspective. J Law Med Ethics 2002;30:594-607.

10. Green S, Davis C, Karshmer E, Marsh P, Straight B. Living Stigma: The Impact of Labeling, Stereotyping, Separation, Status Loss, and Discrimination in the Lives of Individuals with Disabilities and Their Families. Sociol Inq 2005;75:197-215.

11. Parison J, Speare R & Canyon DV (unpublished). Emotional reactions to head lice: results of an internet survey. Available from first author: Julie.Parison@jcu.edu.au

12. Haralambos M, van Krieken R, Smith P, Holborn M. Sociology themes and perspectives (Australian edition). South Melbourne, Victoria: Longman; 1996.

13. Goffman E. Stigma Notes on the Management of Spoiled Identity. Ringwood, Victoria: Penguin Books; 1963.

14. Zinsser H. Rats, lice and history. New York: Bantam; 1960.

15. Douglas M. Purity and Danger - An analysis of concept of pollution and taboo. London: Routledge Classics; 1961.

16. Trigger DS. Blackfellows, whitefellows, and head lice. Australian Institute of Aboriginal Studies Newsletter 1981;15:63-72.

17. Maunder B. Attitude to Head Lice – A More Powerful Force Than Insecticides. J R Soc Health 1985;2:61-64.

18. Heukelbach J, van Haeff E, Rump B, Wilcke T, Moura RC, Feldmeier H. Parasitic skin diseases: health care-seeking in a slum in north-east Brazil. Trop Med Int Health 2003;8:368-373.

19. Kleinman A. Patients and Healers in the Context of Culture. Los Angeles (CA): University of California Press, 1980.

Knowledge and Practices of Health Professionals Regarding Head Lice

8. Knowledge and Practices of Health Professionals Regarding Head Lice

According to the recently published international guidelines on the control of head louse infestations [1], health providers such as physicians, nurses and pharmacists should be knowledgeable about the biology of head lice and the ways to control them effectively. However, there are only few studies available assessing these aspects of head lice control. Philips et al. [2] assessed the general acceptance when pharmacists provide advice and treatment against head lice to parents, in the absence of a referral from general practice nurses or physicians. Direct referral to the pharmacist was shown to be resource saving, due to the lower cost of a pharmacy consultation, as compared to a visit to a general practitioner. However, approximately 52% of patients found it embarrassing or upsetting to ask the pharmacist for advice, while 26.5% were also upset by having to use a louse comb to prove infestation. Increasing confidentiality and privacy within pharmacies may further increase the acceptance of the pharmacy-based approach. Considering the role of pharmacists in giving advice to patients, parents and the community regarding head louse infestations, it was suggested that greater effort should be invested in their education regarding diagnosis and control of head lice infestation. The opinion of health professionals was in general positive regarding this approach. General Practitioners and school nurses noted the positive effect of sparing time usually spent with head lice patients. However, pharmacists stated having problems in explaining the importance of proof of infestations which now need to be done by patients themselves [2].

In a study conducted in South Staffordshire health district, UK, Olowokure et al. [3] examined the knowledge and practice of pediatricians, general practitioners and nurses regarding prevention and treatment of head louse infestations. Eighteen months after dissemination of local guidelines, a questionnaire was sent to the health professionals. Whereas 87% of community health care workers and 74% of health care professionals referred to these guidelines when asked by a patient about head lice, only 43% of pharmacists did so. A considerable number of professionals did not have any knowledge on prevention and treatment of head lice. Only 5% of health care professionals had full knowledge of treatment. In general, knowledge regarding prevention methods was better than knowledge of treatment methods [3]. However, this study presented relative frequencies in a confusing manner and did not define clearly outcome measures such as "poor knowledge", which limits its interpretation.

In another study conducted in Israel, a questionnaire was sent to physicians assessing their knowledge on biology and epidemiology of lice, their clinical experience with infested individuals, and their preferences for diagnosis, prophylaxis and control [4]. Out of 273 physicians, 98 were pediatricians, 66 family physicians, 52 general practitioners and 49 dermatologists, while the remaining 8 were specialists in other medical areas or did not indicate their medical field. An anonymous questionnaire with 37 questions was sent to the private address of physicians, distributed among physicians participating in a dermatological congress or by publishing on a website for physicians in Israel. The results were surprising: In total, 63% of the physicians did not know that head lice cannot jump from head to head, and 60% did not know that lice can survive only for 1-2 days outside their human hosts; 76% knew that lice cannot be transmitted from pets such as dogs and cats to humans. Seventy-one percent did not know that all developmental stages of lice are blood-feeders, while only 63% knew that lice do not feed on dander and sweat. Only 66% knew that head lice do not transmit diseases. The majority of physicians (91%) answered correctly that lice infest children with any length and color of hair. Only 62% of physicians knew that the presence of nits alone is not an accurate indicator of an active head louse infestation and 81% that pruritus is the most common clinical symptom accompanying a louse infestation.

Two-thirds of the physicians correctly stated that a louse comb is the best means for detecting an infestation. In fact, combing the dry hair with a louse comb is four times more effective for the diagnosis of louse infestation and twice as fast as physical examination by hand (☞ also Chapter 5.1.) [5]. The distinction between living lice and nits is especially important as living lice indicate active infestation while nits may only indicate past, non-active infestation without any risk for transmission.

Eighty-four percent of the physicians knew correctly that a second treatment after 7-10 days is usually necessary to control lice, and the vast majority (97%) knew that the louse comb should be an integral part of any anti-louse treatment modality.

Three-quarters of the responders believed that it is the duty of parents to examine their children for lice. Less believed is the responsibility of school nurses (34%) or physicians (23%), but the majority of (88%) believed that head lice are a public health problem. Only 62% perceived that the presence of lice may create psychological and emotional problems in the family. The psychological effects of a louse infestation often exceed the physical ones. Parents, teachers, kindergarten staff, social workers and even nurses and physicians are sometimes distressed by the presence of lice. They often incorrectly blame the child and make him/her feel responsible for the infestation and cause significant damage to the self-esteem of a young child and probably also to his/her parents [6].

Regarding treatment, 63% of the health professionals recommended malathion-containing pediculicides, and 37% recommend anti-louse products containing permethrin. Practically all physicians knew that not all pediculicides on the market are effective and that lice can develop resistance to pediculicides, while only 58% knew that due to its toxic side-effects kerosene alone or in combination with vinegar and oil should not be used for the control of lice and that it is not necessary to treat the environment and the house when lice are detected on inhabitants (87%). Interestingly, several studies from Israel showed that local head lice strains developed resistance to permethrin and cross-resistance to phenothrin [7]. Accordingly, the use of such pediculicides should be avoided. Only about one quarter of the responders recommended that parents use a louse comb for the treatment, while another quarter also recommended natural, which lack authorisation to be sold as pediculicides by health authorities.

Only 2 physicians had a very poor knowledge (1-7 correct answers) and were excluded from analysis, while about 2/3 of the remaining had some knowledge, and 1/3 a good knowledge on pediculosis. Level of knowledge of physicians, according to specialty, is detailed in Table 8.1.

	n	Good knowledge (%)	Some knowledge (%)
Family physician	66	36.4	63.6
Paediatrician	98	40.8	59.2
Dermatologist	49	22.4	77.6
General practitioner	52	25.0	75.0

Table 8.1: Level of knowledge on louse biology, diagnosis, prophylaxis and control among the different groups of physicians.

Paediatricians (83.5%) and dermatologists (93.7%) had examined more frequently at least on child with head lice than family physicians (76.9%) and general practitioners (61.5%).

About half of the physicians believed that they did not have sufficient knowledge to effectively diagnose a louse infestation, while about ¾ believed that they are able to treat an infested individual once lice are detected.

In conclusion, knowledge of health professionals regarding head lice infestations is insufficient, which can be considered one of the major drawbacks in control of pediculosis.

8.1. References

1. Mumcuoglu KY, Barker SC, Burgess IF, Combescot-Lang C, Dagleish RC, Larsen KS, Miller J, Roberts RJ, Taylan-Ozkan A. International guidelines for effective control of head louse infestations. J Drugs Dermatol 2007;6:409-14.

2. Philips Z, Whynes D, Parnham S, Slack R, Earwicker S. The role of community pharmacists in prescribing medication for the treatment of head lice. J Public Health Med 2001;23:114-20.

3. Olowokure B, Jenkinson H, Beaumont M, Duggal HV. The knowledge of healthcare professionals with regard to the treatment and prevention of head lice lice. Int J Env Health Res 2003;13:11-5.

4. Mumcuoglu KY, Mumcuoglu M, Danilevich M, Gilead L. Physician's knowledge in Israel on the biology

and control of head lice (in Hebrew). Harefuah 2008; 147:754-7.

5. Mumcuoglu KY, Friger M, Ioffe-Uspensky I, Ben-Ishai F, Miller J. Louse comb versus direct visual examination for the diagnosis of head louse infestations. Pediatr Dermatol 2001;18:9-12.

6. Mumcuoglu KY. Head lice in drawings of kindergarten children. Isr J Psychiatry Relat Sci 1991;28:25-32.

7. Mumcuoglu KY, Hemingway J, Miller J, Ioffe-Uspensky I, Klaus S, Ben-Ishai F, Galun R. Permethrin resistance in the head louse *Pediculus capitis* from Israel. Med Vet Entomol 1995;9:427-32.

Prevention and Control

9. Prevention and Control

9.1. Control of head lice in developed market economies

In developed market economies pediculosis causes angst which is far out of proportion to its clinical significance. Control has used a biomedical approach, based on the biology of head lice, dispelling myths with evidence and unifying recommendations. Topical insecticides have been the major intervention until the last decade when use of hair conditioner and physical removal of lice using fine tooth combs has been promoted. However, the anxiety provoked by head lice in developed market economies has not been addressed in a systematic way at the population level. Since the socio-emotional area is arguably the major impact of pediculosis in developed market economies, failure to deal with this aspect is a major deficiency in control strategies. The most prominent differences between head lice control in developing countries and developed market economies are that in the former emotional reactions to head lice are far less important.

The major target population in developed market economies is children of primary school age, 6-12 years. Health education and promotion is directed primarily to their parents and guardians. The key settings for increased risk of transmission are primary schools, the family and to a lesser degree, day care centres.

Control of head lice in schools and day care settings is based on health education, early diagnosis (e.g., by screening) and prompt treatment of infested individuals. The activities should be done on a regular basis, as most schools have, at any point in time, children with head lice since prevalence is typically 10% or greater [1, 2]. School based programs typically come either from the government (local or state) or from the school community, particularly parents' associations. However, the government's role in these programs has tended to decline quite markedly in developed market economies, and is now largely one of providing "expert" advice. Some school based programs have been successful in reducing prevalence in smaller primary schools. Typically, intensity of infestation as measured by number of lice per infested child falls dramatically (95%) after a school-wide treatment program, but the prevalence declines by much less (50%) (R. Speare, personal observation). A school based program repeated three times a year seems unable to eliminate head lice from the children, but it can keep the intensity low and maintain prevalence of pediculosis at 10% or less (R. Speare, personal observation). On the other hand, according to the American Academy of Pediatrics, routine screening for nits and lice by school nurses is not considered an effective means to control head lice [3]. The basis for this is that the amount of time and human resources required for screening and the low sensitivity of visual census does not justify the benefits.

9.1.1. Prevention and health education

Evidence-based information should be provided to school staff and parents regularly, irrespective of the prevalence of head lice in the school (☞ Table 9.1). Head lice alert letters about an "outbreak in school" sent by school staff are not recommended, as they increase anxiety, stigma, produce unnecessary public alarm and inappropriate prophylactic treatment by some parents [4]. It should be made clear to school teachers and parents that head lice are not associated with poor hygiene habits, that they do not pose a major health risk and do not transmit any diseases (☞ Table 9.1). Itching is the most common symptom, but is unreliable as an indicator of infestation since it has low sensitivity and specificity. Thus, all family members should check their status by detection combing. The use of repellents to prevent individual infestation is not recommended, as the evidence on effectiveness is deficient [5]. Table 9.1 summarises points to be raised in information leaflets for parents and school staff.

Unfortunately, the advice provided to parents is often contradictory since it comes from multiple "authoritative" sources. Much is not evidence-based and is confusing for lay persons. Information from web sites, product labels, pharmacists, information sheets and media is inconsistent. Advice often erroneously includes treatment of possible fomites such as washing all brushes, combs, ribbons,

9.1. Control of head lice in developed market economies

Clinical aspects
• Most individuals with head lice do not have any symptoms
• When symptoms occur, people usually have been infested for several weeks
• Do not worry too much about head lice—they are a nuisance, but do not transmit any diseases or cause serious harm
• There is no need to feel ashamed because of head lice or to hide an infestation
Diagnosis
• Diagnosis of active head lice infestation can only be made if live lice are found on the scalp
• Diagnosis should be based on detection combing rather than visual inspection
• Adults also get head lice
Transmission
• Head lice are transmitted by direct head-to-head contact
• Head lice do not jump or fly, but may be flicked off by static electricity after dry combing
• You do not get head lice from objects, and transmission via shared objects is very unlikely
• Many infestations occur in families and in the community, besides transmission in schools
• Tracking down the source of head lice can be difficult. Concentrate on opportunities for head to head contact
• Anyone can get lice—it is not an issue of hygiene
• Only humans get head lice—animals do not transmit head lice

Prevention
• Head lice always occur, but there are some periods in the year when incidence is higher
• Exclusion from school will not help in head lice control and is discriminatory
• Check the heads of all family members by detection combing
• Transmission from the environment and objects does not play a role, and treatment of these items is not necessary
• To control head lice concentrate on the head; do not waste time and effort cleaning the house
• The use of repellents is not recommended since there is no evidence they work
• Dead eggs and empty egg shells will remain after treatment and the presence of nits alone does not pose any transmission risk
• Use detection combing once a week 52 weeks of the year
Treatment
• Treatment should only be done if living lice are found and should not be based on the presence of nits
• Most insecticidal treatments require a second treatment after one week
• If the problem continues after treatment, ask advice from local pharmacist or general practitioner
• To prevent reinfestation always synchronise detection combing and treatment in children that have head to head contact
• Do not use products not licensed for treatment of head lice
• Never blame or punish a child for having head lice

Table 9.1: Issues to be raised in information leaflets about managing head lice infestations.

scrunchies, pillowslips and recently worn clothes, or environmental interventions such as vacuum-cleaning furniture, carpeting, car seats and other fabric-covered items, or seal items in bags for two weeks [6, 7]. There is also no need to treat items such as helmets and headphones with insecticide sprays available on the market. In fact, there is no clear evidence that fomites play a significant role in head lice transmission [8-10], and the above described annoying, time-consuming and stressing procedures are not necessary. A list of evidence-based web sites with reliable information can be found in Chapter 12.

9.1.2. Treatment

Treatment should be initiated as soon as possible, but only after confirmation of diagnosis (live head lice found). The selection of treatment should be based on several criteria, such as the local resistance situation, efficacy against lice and eggs, safety, easy application, accessibility and cost (☞ Chapter 6.13.). The philosophy of the parents also plays a significant role since parents are often reluctant to use insecticides whether considered safe or not [11]. In many schools, permethrin and malathion resistance has been observed, which renders the use of these pediculicides ineffective (☞ Chapter 6.4.). In the last years, several options have emerged with no or very low probability of development of resistance, such as silicone oils and ivermectin (☞ Chapters 6.6., 6.8. and 6.9.).

9.1.3. Involvement of stakeholders

For effective control of pediculosis at the population level, collaboration of all stakeholders involved, particularly parents and school teachers, is important [12-15]. The 2008 update of the UK Stafford Report [4] recommended the following responsibilities of the different stakeholders in the control of head lice:

- Parents: Identification, treatment and prevention of head lice in the family. Parents cannot be expected to distinguish current from previous infestation.
- Primary health care professionals: Diagnosis, management and treatment of individuals. Advice and support on treatment and prevention.
- Pharmacists: Should be updated on local policies and protocols and be able to give accurate information to the public. Teach parents the technique of detection combing and advise on appropriate treatment.
- School Health Services: School nurses should provide professional advice to staff, parents and children. Local policies should be carried out and accurate information on head lice provided, independent from the outbreak situation in the school. Teach detection combing to children, parents and staff. Give advice on treatment and prevention. School nurses should not screen pupils on a routine screening basis.
- Head teachers: Collaborate with school nurse and adhere to local protocol. Alert letters should not be sent.

In the UK, the so-called Health Protection Team (consisting of the consultant in communicable disease control, health protection nurse and staff) is responsible for advising about control of head lice in the population as a whole, training school and community nurses, and for producing guidelines for all stakeholders involved [4]. The Health Visitors, which are community workers visiting families with children under five years, should offer advice on detection and treatment of head lice, considering the special aspects of treatment in small children [4].

In some countries, such as in Germany, parents are instructed by law to inform the school or kindergarten when they observe head lice in their children and to confirm treatment [16].

9.1.4. The "No Nit Policy" and exclusion from school

The so-called "No Nit Policy" has been a common practice in the past, and is still being advocated by some groups, school districts, health authorities and consumer organisations in high income countries [3, 17-19]. This practice is based on exclusion of a child from school, holiday camp or child care, until no adult lice, nymphs, viable nits and even empty egg casts are detected. The aim of this is to reduce transmission risk by excluding infested individuals from schools and other institutions. In this context, all nits found on the scalp are considered viable eggs. This means in practice that even in the absence of lice, children would be excluded from school, until treated with a pediculicidal agent and all nits are removed or dyed the same colour of the hair so that they cannot be seen.

The presence of eggs close to the scalp cannot be used as a proxy for active head lice infestation or transmission risk. As detailed in Chapter 5.1. (Diagnosis of head lice infestations), only a small percentage of children with eggs close to the scalp actually have an active infestation [20]. Another study suggested that non-infested children were more frequently excluded from school due to pediculosis than infested children, when diagnosis was based on nits [18].

The no nit policies adopted by many institutions should be discontinued (and in fact have already been banned in several countries [4]), as it is unproductive and may lead to unnecessary treatment in most cases, direct and indirect economic loss, absenteeism from school, social distress and isolation, embarrassment, reduced low-esteem, shame and stigma [4, 17, 19]. Often, a child is sent home from school immediately after diagnosis. This does not make a lot of sense, as infestations are usually detected several weeks after arrival—a few hours more in school will not make a difference in terms of transmission, but is important to prevent the negative effects of excluding pupils from schools [3, 19]. In the USA, an estimated 12-24 million school days were lost in 1998 due to the no nit policy [17], with billions of direct and indirect costs involved annually [19]. Parents are often overloaded when their children are kept out of school and cannot go to work, and as a consequence infestations are hidden from the public. Mumcuoglu et al. (2006) even stated that many parents had lost their jobs as a consequence of absenteeism from school, owing to this policy [19]. On the other side, according to Frankowski (2004), the no nit policy is difficult to explain why it is not effective, especially to lay persons and particularly when consumer organisations support them enthusiastically [3]. Exclusion from school is also not used for other diseases and conditions with low transmissibility such as verrucae or herpes simplex [4].

9.1.5. Conclusion

For effective control of head lice in institutional settings, the collaboration of parents, teachers and healthcare professionals is needed. Early diagnosis is crucial which can be achieved by screening programs in collaboration with parents. If all children at risk or their parents performed diagnostic combing (ideally wet combing with conditioner), head lice would become a minor problem. All family members of infested children should check their infestation status. Considering treatment, the local resistance situation of neurotoxic insecticides should be taken into account. Treatment should only be started when live lice are detected. Environmental measures are ineffective to control head lice in these settings. The no nit policy should be discontinued, as it is contraproductive and causes more harm than good. Exclusion from school cannot ensure elimination of infestation from the family of a child, and in addition is an unproductive and undesirable overreaction to a condition that is not a dangerous health threat [4]. *"No child should lose valuable school time because of head lice"* [19].

9.1.6. References

1. Counahan M, Andrews R, Buttner P, Byrnes G, Speare R. Head lice prevalence in primary schools in Victoria, Australia. J Paediatr Child Health 2004;40:616-619.

2. Speare R, Buettner PG. Head lice in pupils of a primary school in Australia and implications for control. Int J Dermatol 1999;38:285-290.

3. Frankowski BL. American Academy of Pediatrics guidelines for the prevention and treatment of head lice infestation. Am J Man Care 2004; 10:S269-272.

4. Head lice: evidence-based guidelines based on the Stafford Report - 2008 update. Public Health Medicine Environmental Group; 2008.

5. Canyon DV, Speare R. A comparison of botanical and synthetic substances commonly used to prevent head lice (*Pediculus humanus* var. *capitis*) infestation. Int J Dermatol 2007;46:422-426.

6. Frankowski BL, Weiner LB. Head lice. Pediatrics 2002; 110:638-643.

7. Medicines Evaluation Committee. A review of the regulation of head lice treatments in Australia: Australian Government - Department of Health and Ageing - Therapeutic Goods Administration; 2003.

8. Speare R, Cahill C, Thomas G. Head lice on pillows, and strategies to make a small risk even less. Int J Dermatol 2003;42:626-629.

9. Canyon DV, Speare R, Muller R. Spatial and kinetic factors for the transfer of head lice (*Pediculus capitis*) between hairs. J Invest Dermatol 2002;119:629-631.

10. Speare R, Thomas G, Cahill C. Head lice are not found on floors in primary school classrooms. Aust N Z J Public Health 2002;26: 208-211.

11. Parison JC, Speare R, Canyon D. Uncovering family experiences with head lice: the difficulties of eradication. The Open Dermatology Journal 2008;2:9-17.

12. Sarov B, Neumann L, Herman Y, Naggan L. Evaluation of an intervention program for head lice infestation in school children. Pediatr Infect Dis J 1988;7:176-179.

13. Paredes SS, Estrada R, Alarcon H, Chavez G, Romero M, Hay R. Can school teachers improve the management and prevention of skin disease? A pilot study based on head louse infestations in Guerrero, Mexico. Int J Dermatol. 1997;36:826-830.

14. Willems S, Lapeere H, Haedens N, Pasteels I, Naeyaert JM, De Maeseneer J. The importance of socioeconomic status and individual characteristics on the prevalence of head lice in schoolchildren. Eur J Dermatol 2005;15:387-392.

15. Koch T, Brown M, Selim P, Isam C. Towards the eradication of head lice: literature review and research agenda. J Clin Nurs 2001;10:364-371.

16. Epidemiologisches Bulletin Nr. 20/2007. RKI-Ratgeber Infektionskrankheiten. Merkblätter für Ärzte. Kopflausbefall (Pediculosis capitis): Robert-Koch-Institut; 2007.

17. Donnelly E, Lipkin J, Clore ER, Altschuler DZ. Pediculosis prevention and control strategies of community health and school nurses: a descriptive study. J Community Health Nurs 1991;8:85-95.

18. Pollack RJ, Kiszewski AE, Spielman A. Overdiagnosis and consequent mismanagement of head louse infestations in North America. Pediatr Infect Dis J 2000;19:689-693.

19. Mumcuoglu KY, Meinking TA, Burkhart CN, Burkhart CG. Head louse infestations: the "no nit" policy and its consequences. Int J Dermatol 2006;45:891-896.

20. Williams LK, Reichert A, MacKenzie WR, Hightower AW, Blake PA. Lice, nits, and school policy. Pediatrics 2001;107:1011-1015.

9.2. Control of head lice in resource-poor communities

In resource-poor communities throughout the world head lice have considerable public health relevance. In these communities individuals of all age groups are affected. Prevalence in the general population can be up to 40%, and school-age children bear a high burden of disease [1, 2]. Incidence and the probability that most of the household members are infested increase with poverty [2-6].

Considering the low risk of transmission through fomites and the absence of an animal reservoir, theoretically the control of head lice infestation should not be a difficult task. However, control strategies must be adapted to the setting and those recommended so far are usually not evidence-based [7-10]. The presence of more important health hazards in resource-poor settings, neglect and ignorance of the population are reasons why head lice control usually is not on the agenda of policy makers and health care providers. This is of concern, as in affected communities head lice infestations are associated with high morbidity [1, 6, 11, 12].

Community control of head lice is feasible, if based on mass treatment and health education. Treatment of the environment and of fomites is not necessary. Ideally, mass treatment is done with ivermectin (200 µg/kg body weight, two doses 8-10 days apart), a highly effective oral drug with the additional benefit that it acts against intestinal helminths, scabies and cutaneous larva migrans (☞ Chapter 6.8. for details) [13-15]. Mass administration of ivermectin reduced the prevalence of active head lice infestation in the general population from 16% to 1% in a resource-poor fishing community in northeast Brazil [13]. After nine months, prevalence of pediculosis was still significantly lower (10%) than before intervention.

Due to its favourable safety profile, we recommend treatment of all individuals in an endemic community >5 years independent of their infestation status, excluding pregnant and breastfeeding women who may be treated with a topical pediculicide. The intervention should be repeated 1-2 times per year. Ivermectin has been used in millions of individuals in onchocerciasis and lymphatic filariasis control programs and is considered safe for community treatment [14, 16, 17].

Mass treatment with topically applicable neurotoxic pediculicides such as permethrin is not recommended in resource-poor communities. This approach needs more health education and requires substantial human resources. There is always the risk that the compound is not used correctly which poses a health hazard and bears the risk of inducing resistant lice populations [7, 10, 18]. In countries where ivermectin is not available at low cost, a better alternative is the application of silicone-based pediculicides with a physical mode of action (dimeticone). These compounds are safe, culturally acceptable, effective and do not bear the risk of developing resistance (☞ Chapter 6.6. for details).

A recent randomised trial has shown the importance of intra-familiar and peri-domiciliar community transmission in resource-poor settings, further highlighting the importance of mass treatment of the general population, rather than treatment of single individuals [3]. In 132 head lice-free children from a slum in northeast Brazil, incidence of head lice infestations was determined in an intervention group (treatment of all family members with oral ivermectin, excluding study participants) and a control group (family members untreated). Children in the intervention group remained significantly longer without infestation with a median infestation-free time of 24 days, as compared to 14 days in the control group (p=0.03; ☞ Figure 9.1).

Health education should accompany campaigns of mass treatment and be adapted to local concepts of the disease, focussing on the most vulnerable population groups, typically children and mothers.

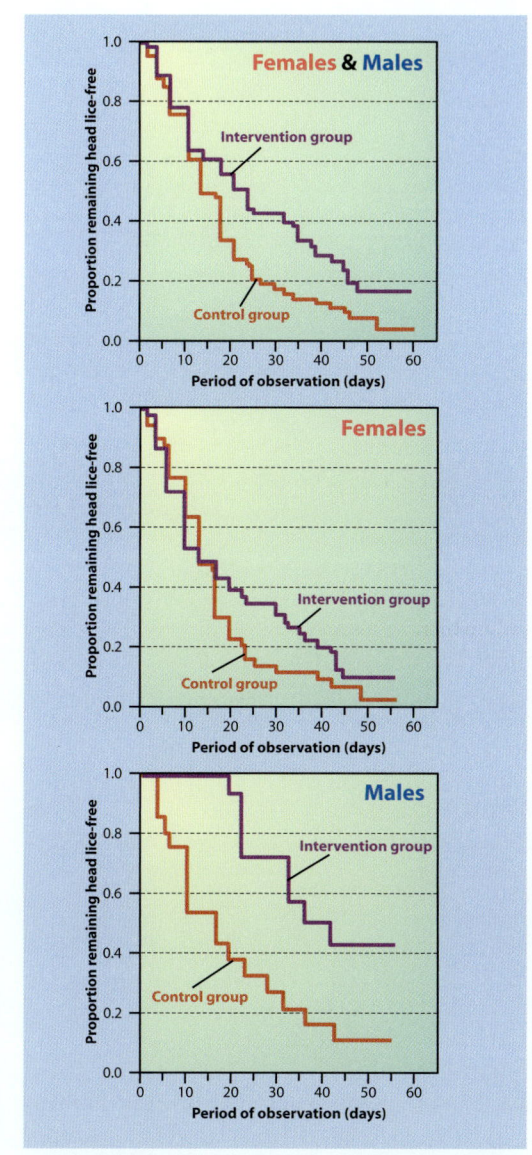

Figure 9.1: Head-lice free periods of individuals living in an endemic area in Brazil (total population and stratified by gender). In the intervention group, family members were treated with oral ivermectin (reproduced from Pilger et al. 2010 [3]).

9.2.1. References

1. Heukelbach J, Wilcke T, Winter B, Feldmeier H. Epidemiology and morbidity of scabies and pediculosis capitis in resource-poor communities in Brazil. Br J Dermatol 2005;153:150-156.

2. Bachok N, Nordin RB, Awang CW, Ibrahim NA, Naing L. Prevalence and associated factors of head lice infestation among primary schoolchildren in Kelantan, Malaysia. Southeast Asian J Trop Med Public Health 2006;37:536-543.

3. Pilger D, Heukelbach J, Khakban A, Oliveira FA, Fengler G, Feldmeier H. Impact of household-wide treatment for the control of head lice infestations in an impoverished community: randomized observer-blinded comparative trial. Bull World Health Organ 2010;88:90-96.

4. Amr ZS, Nusier MN. Pediculosis capitis in northern Jordan. Int J Dermatol 2000;39:919-921.

5. Catala S, Junco L, Vaporaky R. Pediculus capitis infestation according to sex and social factors in Argentina. Rev Saude Publica 2005;39:438-443.

6. Suleman M, Jabeen N. Head lice infestation in some urban localities of NWFP, Pakistan. Ann Trop Med Parasitol 1989;83:539-547.

7. Heukelbach J, de Oliveira FA, Feldmeier H. Ectoparasitoses and public health in Brazil: challenges for control. Cad Saude Publica 2003;19:1535-1540.

8. Feldmeier H, Heukelbach J. Epidermal parasitic skin diseases: a neglected category of poverty-associated plagues. Bull World Health Organ 2009;87:152-159.

9. Ugbomoiko US, Speare R, Heukelbach J. Self-diagnosis of head lice infestation in rural Nigeria as a reliable rapid assessment tool for pediculosis. The Open Dermatology Journal 2008;2:95-97.

10. Burgess IF. Current treatments for pediculosis capitis. Curr Opin Infect Dis 2009;22:131-136.

11. Feldmeier H, Chhatwal GS, Guerra H. Pyoderma, group A streptococci and parasitic skin diseases —a dangerous relationship. Trop Med Int Health 2005;10:713-716.

12. Heukelbach J, van Haeff E, Rump B, Wilcke T, Moura RC, Feldmeier H. Parasitic skin diseases: health care-seeking in a slum in north-east Brazil. Trop Med Int Health 2003;8:368-373.

13. Heukelbach J, Winter B, Wilcke T, Muehlen M, Albrecht S, Oliveira FA, et al. Selective mass treatment with ivermectin to control intestinal helminthiases and parasitic skin diseases in a severely affected population. Bull World Health Organ 2004;82:563-571.

14. Fox LM. Ivermectin: uses and impact 20 years on. Curr Opin Infect Dis 2006;19:588-593.

15. Lawrence G, Leafasia K, Sheridan J, Hills S, Wate J, Wate C, et al. Control of scabies, skin sores and haematuria in children in the Solomon Islands: another role for ivermectin. Bull World Health Organ 2005;83:34-42.

16. Stephenson I, Wiselka M. Drug treatment of tropical parasitic infections: recent achievements and developments. Drugs 2000;60:985-995.

17. Dourmishev AL, Dourmishev LA, Schwartz RA. Ivermectin: pharmacology and application in dermatology. Int J Dermatol 2005;44:981-988.

18. Sarov B, Neumann L, Herman Y, Naggan L. Evaluation of an intervention program for head lice infestation in school children. Pediatr Infect Dis J 1988;7:176-179.

Regulatory Aspects of Head Lice Products

10. Regulatory Aspects of Head Lice Products

This chapter will look at the different regulatory aspects of head lice products. Because of national variations, we focus on the situation in the European Union.

On a legislative basis, a product to treat head lice infestations can only be a **medicinal product** or a **medical device** because by definition only these two product classes are able to treat diseases in man. Therefore, a pediculicide is in Europe *either* regulated as a medical device by the corresponding Medical Device Directive (MDD 93/42/EEC [1]) *or* as a medicinal product by the corresponding Medicinal Product Directive (MPD 2001/83/EC [2]). The procedure—authorisation or conformity assessment—to be followed prior to placing a product on the market will therefore be governed by the MDD or by the MPD. However, some variations of this rule occur in particular countries.

10.1. Medical devices

■ Step 1 – Categorisation

The first question is: Is the head lice product to be registered a medical device?

Article 1, No. 2 a of the Council Directive 93/42/EEC [1, 3] defines a medical device as *"any instrument, apparatus, appliance, software, material or other article, whether used alone or in combination, including the software intended by its manufacturer to be used specifically for diagnostic and/or therapeutic purposes and necessary for its proper application intended by the manufacturer to be used for human beings for the purpose of:*

- diagnosis, prevention, monitoring, treatment or alleviation of disease,

- diagnosis, monitoring, treatment, alleviation of or compensation for an injury or handicap,

- investigation, replacement or modification of the anatomy or of a physiological process,

- control of contraception,

and which does not achieve its principal intended action in or on the human body by pharmacological, immunological or metabolic means, but which may be assisted in its function by such means."

Thus, if the pediculicide kills lice by physical or physico-chemical means, it has to be categorised as a medical device.

■ Step 2 – Classification

The next question would be: The medical device does belong to which risk class?

Devices are classified according to risk, duration of application, invasiveness, technology and intended use as described in the classification rules (Annex IX of the MDD 93/42/EEC).

The design of the device has to reflect the potential risk associated with the device. The higher the risk and the risk class, respectively, the more efforts are required to minimise the risk. Thus, the most stringent precautions are required for those devices which present the highest risks to health or safety.

Four different risk classes are defined:

- Class I for low-risk devices
- Class IIa and IIb for medium-risk devices
- Class III for high-risk devices

In the European Union medical devices against head lice infestations are usually classified as class I devices. However, the German competent authorities have decided that medical devices against pediculosis are classified as IIa devices.

■ Step 3 – Access to the Market

The final question is: Which requirements must be fulfilled to allow access to the market for the medical device?

▶ Essential Requirements

All medical devices must fulfil the Essential Requirements in respect of safety owed to patients, users and other personnel, efficacy and quality. These Essential Requirements are defined in Annex I of the MDD 93/42/EEC and state that:

- the device must be designed and manufactured in such a way that, when used under the conditions and purposes intended, it will not compromise the health or safety of patients, users or other personnel
- safety principles must be utilised for the design and construction, and it should include state-of-the-art technologies

10.1. Medical devices

- the device must meet all claimed performance criteria
- the device must continue to function as intended, without compromising safety or health, when subjected to normal conditions of use
- the device should not be adversely affected during defined transport and storage conditions
- any undesirable side effects must constitute an acceptable risk when weighed against intended performance

▶ Design and construction requirements

The detailed requirements of Annex I define a variety of design requirements to be met (as applicable), including:

- Chemical, physical and biological properties
- Prevention of microbial contamination
- Construction and environmental properties
- Properties for devices with a measuring function
- Protection against radiation
- Protection against electrical, mechanical, thermal risks, energy supplies
- Labelling requirements and instructions for use
- Demonstration of conformance with essential requirements based on clinical data

With the Directive 2007/47/EC changes to the MDD 93/42/EEC are implemented which have impact on medical devices and their responsible manufacturer, e.g. clarification that each medical device needs to be supported by clinical data and a clinical evaluation (Directive 2007/47/EC [3]). This aspect was not clearly formulated in the MDD 93/42/EEC, a fact that was exploited by some manufacturers by marketing products with insufficient or completely missing clinical data.

▶ Conformity Assessment Procedures
(Article 11 of the MDD 93/42/EEC)

The compliance with the Essential und other legal requirements is evaluated in a conformity assessment procedure, also called certification procedure. The mode and the extent of such a procedure depend on the risk class of the respective device. The higher the risk the lower is the self responsibility of the manufacturer (☞ Figure 10.1).

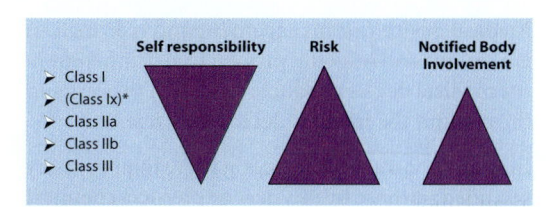

Figure 10.1: Impact of the risk (class) to the self responsibility of the manufacturer and the Notified Body Involvement.
* Class I devices with measuring function (e.g. measuring cup) or sterile devices.

For Class I devices the certification procedure is done by the manufacturer alone. For all other risk classes the participation of a Notified Body is mandatory. Medical devices of the risk classes Ix to III have a CE marking with the identification number of the participating Notified Body. Notified Bodies are certification bodies, appointed by the EU member states.

▶ CE marking

The CE marking is a mandatory European marking for certain product groups, such as medical devices, to indicate conformity with the essential requirements set out in European Directives (e.g. MDD 93/42/EEC), and must be affixed on the device by the legally responsible manufacturer. If a medical device is CE marked it can be sold in all member states of the European Economic Area and Turkey if the labelling and the Instructions for Use are presented in the particular national language.

▶ Risk management

"Risk" is defined as *"combination of the probability of occurrence of harm and the severity of that harm."* (ISO 14971 : 2007 [4])

"Medical device risk management" is defined as *"systematic application of management policies, procedures and practices, to the tasks of analysing, evaluating, monitoring and controlling risk."* (ISO 14971 : 2007 [4])

It is acknowledged that "absolute safety" in medical devices is unattainable; however, the standard ISO 14971: 2007 [4] describes and recommends management policies, procedures and practices of a system to analyse, evaluate and control risk. A medical device risk management process is required as a component of the design of a medical device.

Medical device risk management and risk analysis is a serious and ongoing process that is inherent in the medical device product realisation process and throughout the medical device life cycle.

In summary, medical devices achieve their primary intended purpose by physical or physico-chemical means, are classified according to the risk profile of the product, are supposed to fulfill the Essential Requirements regarding safety, efficacy and quality, must pass through the adequate Conformity Assessment Procedure, have to be CE-marked, and require an ongoing risk management process.

10.2. Medicinal products

10.2.1. Legal requirements

A medicinal product is defined as *"any substance or combination of substances presented as having properties for treating or preventing disease in human beings; or as any substance or combination of substances which may be used in or administered to human beings either with a view to restoring, correcting or modifying physiological functions by exerting a pharmacological, immunological or metabolic action, or to making a medical diagnosis."* (Article 1, No. 2, Directive 2001/83/EC of the European Parliament and of the Council as amended [2])

Within the European Economic Area (EEA), a medicinal product may only be placed on the market when a marketing authorisation (MA) has been issued. The most important criterion for granting a marketing authorisation is the risk-benefit ratio. After demonstrating with stipulated documents on efficacy, safety and pharmaceutical quality that potential risks are outweighed by the therapeutic efficacy, a MA will be assigned. If the risk-benefit-ratio becomes negative after assignation of a MA, the medicinal product must be taken off the market.

In cases of doubt, if a product may fall within the definition of a "medicinal product" or a "medical device", the provisions of the Medicinal Product Directive apply.

■ **Marketing Authorisation Procedures**

Within the EEA there are different MA procedures a pharmaceutical entrepreneur may choose [6] (☞ Figure 10.2).

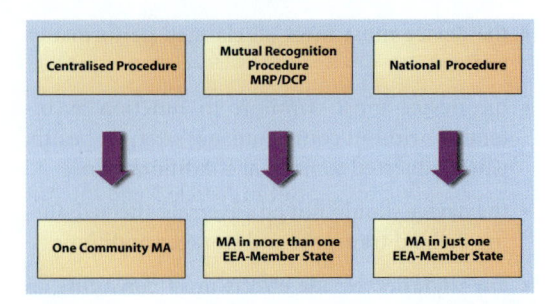

Figure 10.2: Marketing Authorisation Procedures in the EEA.

All different MA procedures have in common that the applications have to be accompanied by a detailed documentation, submitted in accordance with Directive 2001/83/EC. The following information has to be given (the list is not exhaustive):

- Name and permanent address of the applicant and the manufacturer
- Qualitative and quantitative particulars of all the constituents of the medicinal product
- Particulars of the medicinal product: name, pharmaceutical form, method and route of administration, therapeutic indications, contraindications, adverse reactions, posology and expected shelf life
- Reasons for any precautionary and safety measures to be taken for the storage of the medicinal product, and its administration to patients
- Evaluation of the potential environmental risks posed by the medicinal product
- Description of the manufacturing method
- Description of the control methods
- Results of pharmaceutical (physico-chemical, biological or microbiological) tests, pre-clinical (toxicological and pharmacological) tests, and clinical trials
- A detailed description of the pharmacovigilance and, where appropriate, of the risk-management system which the applicant will introduce
- A summary of the product characteristics, a mock-up of the outer packaging, and of the immediate packaging of the medicinal product, and a package leaflet

▶ Centralised procedure

Regulation (EC) No 726/2004 lays down a centralised Community procedure for the authorisation of medicinal products, for which there is a single application, a single evaluation, a single prescription status, a single name and a single authorisation allowing direct access to the single market of the Community.

The types of products which fall within the scope of the Regulation are set out in Article 3 and the Annex to that Regulation. For instance, the use of the centralised procedure is obliged for medicinal products developed by means of specific biotechnological processes (e.g. recombinant DNA technology or hybridoma and monoclonal antibody methods) as well as for medicinal products containing a new active substance to treat acquired immune deficiency syndrome, cancer, neurodegenerative disorders, diabetes, auto-immune diseases and other immune dysfunctions, or viral diseases.

Any medicinal product may be granted a marketing authorisation by the Community on request of the applicant, if the medicinal product contains a new active substance which, on the date of entry into force of Regulation (EC) No 726/2004, was not authorised in the Community; or the applicant shows that the medicinal product constitutes a significant therapeutic, scientific or technical innovation or that the granting of a Community authorisation is in the interests of patients at Community level.

The scientific evaluation of the application is carried out within the Committee for Medicinal Products for Human Use (CHMP) of the European Medicines Agency (EMEA), and a scientific opinion is prepared. Based on this opinion the European Commission drafts a Decision. Having consulted the Member States through the relevant Standing Committee, the Commission adopts the decision and grants a marketing authorisation [5, 8, 9].

▶ (Independent) national procedure

Independent national procedures are limited from 1 January 1998 to medicinal products which are not to be authorised in more than one Member State and to the initial phase of mutual recognition (granting of the marketing authorisation by the Reference Member State).

▶ Mutual recognition procedure (MRP)/ Decentralised procedure (DCP)

The mutual recognition procedure and decentralised procedure must be used for applications for marketing authorisation for medicinal products in more than one Member State with the exception of those medicinal products which are subject to the centralised procedure. The legal provisions are embodied in Directive 2001/83/EC.

- *Mutual recognition procedure (MRP)*
  If a national marketing authorisation for a medicinal product has been granted in one Member State and for which an application is planned to be submitted in other Member States an MRP must be initiated by the holder of the MA.

- *Decentralised procedure (DCP)*
  In cases where no marketing authorisation has been granted in the Community, the applicant should use the DCP and submit an application in all Member States where he intends to obtain a marketing authorisation at the same time, and choose one of them as reference Member State.

MRP and DCP are based on the recognition by national competent authorities (Concerned Member States – CMS) of a first assessment performed by the authorities of one Member State (Reference Member State – RMS), unless there are grounds for supposing that the authorisation of the medicinal product concerned may present a potential serious risk to public health. Differences in proposed prescription status and names of the medicinal product are possible, in line with national rules in force [7].

■ **Continuous update of marketing authorisations**

Throughout the life of a medicinal product, the marketing authorisation must be regularly updated in order to ensure that scientific progress and new regulatory requirements are respected. Any information which may influence the evaluation of the risk-benefit-balance of the medicinal product must be given to the competent authorities. In addition, the competent authorities should be informed relating to any pharmacovigilance concerns.

■ **Validity of the marketing authorisation**

Marketing authorisations have an initial duration of five years. After these five years, the marketing authorisation has to be renewed on the basis of a re-evaluation of the risk-benefit balance. After the renewal, the marketing authorisation is valid for an unlimited period unless the Commission or the national competent authority decides, on justified grounds relating to pharmacovigilance, to proceed with one additional five-year renewal.

■ Clinical aspects in regulatory settings

Both, medical devices and medicinal products, need clinical data to support the product certification or marketing authorisation, respectively. Therefore these pediculicides *should* be effective at the moment of first placing on the market. In discrepancy to current official regulations many products without satisfying safety or efficacy data are still on the market and even if a product has been proven to be effective this can change, because living organisms can adapt to their environment and formerly valid and reliable efficacy data may become obsolete.

10.3. Comment

The majority of medicinal products kill lice by means of pharmacologically active ingredients and are thus classified as medicinal products. Most of them contain neurotoxic insecticides as active ingredient, such as pyrethrum extract, synthetic pyrethroids (e.g. allethrin, permethrin), organophosphates (malathion) or carbamates. As a result of their extensive use, resistances to these pediculicides have increased worldwide (☞ Chapter 6.4. for details).

Other concerns regarding these products are associated with the risk of toxic side effects of medicinal products. For example, lindane was phased out in Europe in 2007 because of its unfavourable toxicological and environmental profile.

More recently developed products, such as those based on dimeticones (silicone oils) exhibit a physical mode of action and are thus classified as medical devices in almost all European countries. These products are of special interest for head lice control, because they are regarded non-toxic to humans, and due to their mode of action the development of resistances is unlikely (☞ Chapters 6.6. and 6.13.).

Another group of pediculicides is based on herbal and essential oils. Manufacturers of some products claim a pure physical mode of action, although this is questioned by experts (☞ Chapter 6.7.). Nevertheless, in some countries these products are registered as medical devices. Valid efficacy and safety data of herbal products are often deficient, and many products on the market may not have any considerable efficacy. For example, Heukelbach et al. (2008) recently reported that in a standardised *in vitro* test only one of six tested plant-based head lice products marketed in Australia showed a considerable degree of efficacy against adult head lice [10]. In addition, many herbal products are not sold in child-proof containers. Reports of toxicity in children after accidental ingestion of herbal products show that they only should be sold in child-proof containers with warning labels [11].

The status (medical device or medicinal product), as well as a valid market approval of a head lice product is not a warrantor for its safety or efficacy. Therefore, government regulatory agencies should require standard *in vitro* tests with stringent criteria for the assessment of lice mortality, to determine the efficacy of new as well as already licensed products. National recommendations and guidelines regarding the treatment of head lice should only be based on data of recently performed studies, such as standardised *in vitro* studies as well as randomised clinical trials following the standards of Evidence-Based Medicine. These guidelines should include head lice products independently from their product class, be updated on a regular basis and consider the possibility of resistance.

10.4. References

1. Council Directive 93/42/EEC of 14 June 1993 concerning medical devices.

2. Directive 2001/83/EC of the European Parliament and of the Council of 6 November 2001 on the Community code relating to medicinal products for human use (Consolidated version : 30/12/2008).

3. Directive 2007/47/EC of the European Parliament and of the Council of 5 September 2007 amending Council Directive 90/385/EEC on the approximation of the laws of the Member States relating to active implantable medical devices, Council Directive 93/42/EEC concerning medical devices and Directive 98/8/EC concerning the placing of biocidal products on the market.

4. ISO 14971: 2007 Medical devices - Application of risk management to medical devices.

5. Regulation (EC) No 726/2004 of the European Parliament and of the Council of 31 March 2004 laying down Community procedures for the authorisation and supervision of medicinal products for human and veterinary use and establishing a European Medicines Agency (Consolided version : 6/7/2009).

6. The Rules governing Medicinal Products in the European Community, The Notice to Applicants, Volume 2A Procedures for marketing authorisation, Chapter 1 - Marketing Authorisation, November 2005.

7. The Rules governing Medicinal Products in the European Community, The Notice to Applicants, Volume 2A Procedures for marketing authorisation, Chapter 2 - Mutual Recognition, February 2007.

8. The Rules governing Medicinal Products in the European Community, The Notice to Applicants, Volume 2A Procedures for marketing authorisation, Chapter 4 - Centralised Procedure, April 2006.

9. The Rules governing Medicinal Products in the European Community, The Notice to Applicants, Volume 2A Procedures for marketing authorisation, Chapter 6 - Community Marketing Authorisation, November 2005.

10. Heukelbach J, Canyon DV, Oliveira FA, Muller R, Speare R. *In vitro* efficacy of over-the-counter botanical pediculicides against the head louse *Pediculus humanus* var *capitis* based on a stringent standard for mortality assessment. Med Vet Entomol 2008;22:264-272.

11. Heukelbach J, Canyon D, Speare R. The effect of natural products on head lice: *in vitro* tests and clinical evidence. J Pediatr Inf Dis 2007;2:67-76.

Lice as Vectors of Pathogenic Microorganisms

11. Lice as Vectors of Pathogenic Microorganisms

As detailed in Chapter 2., *Pediculus capitis* and *Pediculus corporis* are two closely related subspecies that parasitise humans for millions of years. Although body lice and head lice have distinct ecologic preferences, they are morphologically indistinguishable by the naked eye. Whether an experienced entomologist can distinguish the two subspecies in a dissecting microscope, is still a matter of debate [1]. In fact, a recent genetic analysis did not find any differences between the two subspecies [2]. As a consequence, in practice head and body lice are differentiated according to the body parts where they are found and not by entomological characteristics.

Since the pioneering work of Nicolle in 1909, an array of human pathogens has been identified in body lice (☞ Table 11.1) [3]. The most notable are *Rickettsia prowazekii*, the causing agent of louse-borne epidemic typhus; *Borrelia recurrentis* causing louse-borne relapsing fever, and *Bartonella quintana*, the causing agent of trench fever, endocarditis and bacillary angiomatosis. In some cases, the role of *P. corporis* as a highly effective vector has been proved in the laboratory as well as under field conditions, for others the evidence is limited to experimental infections (☞ Table 11.1).

As body lice and head lice are biologically similar, it seems plausible that they have the same capacity of transmitting pathogenic microorganisms. However, there is still insufficient evidence on the vector capacity of head lice (☞ Table 11.2). The experiments by Nicolle suggested that the body louse is a vector of *R. prowazekii*, although it was not investigated whether head lice could transmit this pathogen as well [3].

Already in the beginning of the 20th century, Goldberger and Anderson (1912) collected head lice from patients with louse-borne epidemic typhus and used these lice to infect rhesus monkeys with *R. prowazekii* [4]. Their findings were later confirmed by Murray and Torrey (1975), who infected head lice with *R. prowazekii* by feeding them on a rabbit infected with the pathogen [5]. By using labelled antibodies to *R. prowazekii*, they demonstrated that after six days head lice passed infective rickettsiae in faeces. For unknown reasons, these experiments, although rather simple, have never

Pathogen	Transmission proved		Reference
	experimentally	in endemic/epidemic situations	
R. prowazekii	+	+	Raoult and Roux 1999 [9] Fournier et al. 2002 [12]
R. rickettsii	+	−	Houhamdi and Raoult 2006 [16]
R. conorii	+	−	Houhamdi and Raoult 2006 [16]
B. typhi	+	−	Houhamdi et al. 2003 [17]
B. quintana	+	+	Sparrow 1939 [18] Raoult and Roux 1999 [9] Fournier et al. 2002 [12]
B. recurrentis *B. duttoni*	+ +	+ +	Sparrow 1958 [19] Raoult and Roux 1999 [9] Houhamdi and Raoult 2005 [20]
Yersinia pestis	+	(+)[a]	Houhamdi et al. 2006 [21]
Acinetobacter (baumanii, lwoffi)	+	−	La Scola and Raoult 2004 [22] Houhamdi and Raoult 2006 [23]
F. tularensis	(+)[b]	(+)[b]	Raoult and Roux 1999 [9]

Table 11.1: Body lice as vectors of pathogenic microorganisms.
[a] assumably during plague epidemics in Medievial Age, [b] so far, only the rabbit louse (*Haemodipsus ventricosus*) and the mouse louse (*Polyplax serratus*) have been found infected.

Pathogen	Transmission proved		Reference
	experimentally	in endemic/epidemic situations	
R. prowazekii	+	–	Goldberger and Anderson 1912 [4] Murray and Torrey 1975 [5]
B. quintana	–	+	Sasaki et al. 2006 [14] Bonilla et al. 2009 [15]
B. recurrentis	–	–	
Staphylococci, streptococci	+[a]	n.a.	Meinking 1999 [24]

Table 11.2: Head lice as vectors of pathogenic microorganisms.
[a] only passive transfer. n.a. = not applicable.

been repeated, and the role head lice may have in transmission of louse-borne epidemic typhus has never been scrutinised.

Thorough investigations were hindered by two other presumptions: infective faeces of body lice are more likely to build up in clothes than that of head lice in the hair, and body lice are present in large numbers in patients with louse-borne epidemic typhus, but head lice are not. Both beliefs, though, are not correct. In fact, even very small amounts of lice faeces can be infective [6], and faeces of head lice may build up to substantial levels on the scalp, hair and on pillows of infested people [7]. Moreover, the dust-like faeces may facilitate infection via inhalation, through excoriations of the scalp or contact with the conjunctiva [8]. For instance, hospital cleaners with direct contact to patients became infected when changing the linen of patients with louse-borne epidemic typhus, probably by inhaling airborne louse faeces [9].

In addition, in individuals affected by louse-borne epidemic typhus in certain settings such as in the developing world, head lice may be present in large numbers without being noted. For instance, in the 1975 outbreak of louse-borne epidemic typhus in Uganda, lice eggs were found in both hair and clothes of patients, confirming the presence of head lice [8]. Between 1981 and 1990, epidemics in Ethiopian refugee camps accounted for 69% of all reported cases of epidemic typhus in Africa. Head lice were found on 65% of these people, and close to 100% in children, whereas only 30% of individuals examined had body lice [9]. In susceptible populations, head lice can be present in equally or even larger numbers during epidemics of louse-borne typhus as compared to body lice, but they have been ignored in outbreak investigations.

In the aftermath of World War I, an outbreak of louse-borne epidemic typhus occurred in Poland to which the American army responded with an extensive campaign between 1919 and 1920 [8]. Although the aim of the intervention was to eliminate body lice, by providing clean clothing and blankets, the people's heads were also shaved, thereby controlling head lice. Similarly, an outbreak of louse-borne epidemic typhus in a Burundi jail in 1996, attributed to the presence of body lice, was contained with delousing procedures including head-shaving [10]. Finally, an interesting case occurred in 1998, when a man returning from Algeria to France developed louse-borne typhus [11]. No evidence of body lice was found, but the patient did recall having intensive pruritus of the scalp and scratching during his stay in Algeria.

If head lice have the capacity to transmit *R. prowazekii*, why outbreaks of louse-borne epidemic typhus have not been reported in schools, households or other institutions where carriers of head lice are prevalent? Obviously, there are several requirements that *P. capitis* can become a vector of *R. prowazekii*. The pathogen must circulate in the respective population. Hence, the failure to detect *R. prowazekii* in body lice recovered from adults in endemic African countries, but not in head lice collected from school children in France, Portugal, Russia, China, Thailand and Australia [12] may simply indicate that this essential prerequisite was not completed. Second, *R. prowazekii* needs an immunocompromised host for significant bacteraemia to develop, the latter being a prerequisite for the uptake of the pathogen by the vector during blood-feeding. In the characteristic setting of louse-borne epidemic typhus, impaired immunocompetence may have many reasons such as malnutrition, chronic infections or drug use. Typically, individuals at risk, such as prisoners in developing countries, refugees during war times, homeless people or debilitated soldiers usually share several of these characteristics. A classical example of a high risk group are the >100,000 exhausted soldiers of Napoleon's army returning from Moscow in autumn 1812 of which an unknown portion succumbed to louse-borne epidemic typhus [13].

Finally, the number of lice present on an individual infected with *R. prowazekii* must be sufficiently high, so that the pathogen can be detected in at least one louse. This is illustrated by the observation that in 17 epidemic/endemic situations of louse-borne typhus in only four occasions *R. prowazekii* could be isolated from body lice with a highly sensitive PCR [12].

By consequence, head lice could become a vector for louse-borne typhus and cause an epidemic, when the three prerequisites—circulation of *R. prowazekii* in the population, a high density of head lice on the scalp and impaired immunocompetence of the host—occur.

This assumption is convincingly underlined by the identification of the second important pathogen, *B. quintana*, in head lice of Nepalese children and homeless US-American adults. Sasaki et al. (2006) [14] identified *B. quintana* in 0% of head lice recovered from healthy school children living in Pokhara town, Nepal, but in 12.5% of head lice collected from the scalp of street children or from children living in a slum. Body lice were found in 25% and 19% of these cases, respectively. Besides, homeless children were significantly more often co-infested with body and head lice than children from the other groups.

Bonilla et al. (2009) [15] examined 138 homeless adults from San Francisco for the presence of body and head lice; 23.9% of the individuals were infested with body lice, 8.7% with head lice, and 4.3% had co-infestations. *Bartonella* DNA was detected in one third of body lice-infested and in one quarter of head lice-infested persons. When data were compared between pools of lice, the positive-rate for *B. quintana* DNA was 5.0% in body lice and 8.3% in head lice. Since *B. quintana* was identified in head lice from persons without a concurrent body louse infestation, this study demonstrates that *P. capitis* in fact can act as a vector for *B. quintana*.

Due to the very restricted geographical occurrence of *B. recurrentis* (almost exclusively in the Ethiopian highlands) and the scarce epidemiological data on louse-borne relapsing fever, no data exist to conclude whether head lice can transmit also this pathogen. However, based on the assumptions made above, it is conceivable, that *P. capitis* may also act as a vector in louse-borne relapsing fever.

In summary, there is reason to suggest that head lice can transmit the three most important pathogens found in body lice, namely *R. prowazekii*, *B. quintana* and *B. recurrentis*. Provided that essential epidemiological requirements are accomplished, *P. capitis* could play a similar role as *P. corporis* in transmission dynamics in settings characterised by poverty, neglect, deficient hygiene and rudimentary sanitation.

11.1. References

1. Parola P, Fournier PE, Raoult D. *Bartonella quintana*, lice, and molecular tools. J Med Entomol 2006;43:215.

2. Light JE, Toups MA, Reed DL. What's in a name: the taxonomic status of human head and body lice. Mol Phylogenet Evol 2008;47.

3. Gross L. How Charles Nicolle of the Pasteur Institute discovered that epidemic typhus is transmitted by lice: reminiscences from my years at the Pasteur Institute in Paris. Proc Natl Acad Sci USA 1996;93:10539-10540.

4. Goldberger J, Anderson JF. The transmission of typhus fever, with especial reference to transmission by the head louse (*Pediculus capitis*). Public Health Rep 1912:297-307.

5. Murray ES, Torrey SB. Virulence of *Rickettsia prowazekii* for head lice. Ann NY Acad Sci 1975;266:25-34.

6. Buxton PA. The louse - An account of the lice which infest man, their medical importance and control. London: Edward Arnold, 1947.

7. Burgess IF. Human lice and their control. Annu Rev Entomol 2004;49:457-481.

8. Robinson D, Leo N, Prociv P, Barker SC. Potential role of head lice, *Pediculus humanus capitis*, as vectors of *Rickettsia prowazekii*. Parasitol Res 2003;90:209-211.

9. Raoult D & Roux V. The body louse as a vector of reemerging human diseases. Clin Inf Dis 1999;29:888-911.

10. Raoult D, Roux V, Ndihokubwayo JB, Bise G, Baudon D, Martet G et al. Jail fever (epidemic typhus)—Outbreak in Burundi. Emerg Inf Dis 1997;3:357-360.

11. Niang M, Brouqui P, Raoult D. Epidemic typhus imported from Algeria. Emerg Inf Dis 1999;5:716-718.

12. Fournier PE, Ndihokubwayo JB, Guidran J, Kelly PJ, Raoult D. Human pathogens in body and head lice. Emerg Inf Dis 2002;8:1515-1518.

13. Raoult D, Dutour O, Houhamdi L, Jankauskas R, Fournier PE, Ardagna Y et al. Evidence for louse-transmitted diseases in soldiers of Napoleon's grand army in Vilnius. J Inf Dis 2006;193:112-120.

14. Sasaki T, Poudel SKS, Isawa H, Hayashi T, Seki N, Tomita T et al. First Molecular Evidence of *Bartonella quintana* in *Pediculus humanus capitis* (Phthiraptera: Pediculidae), Collected from Nepalese Children. J Med Entomol 2006;43:110-112.

15. Bonilla DL, Kabeya H, Henn J, Kramer VL, Kosoy MY. *Bartonella quintana* in body lice and head lice from homeless persons, San Francisco, California, USA. Emerg Inf Dis 2009;15:912-915.

16. Houhamdi L, Raoult D. Experimentally infected human body lice (*Pediculus humanus humanus*) as vectors of *Rickettsia rickettsii* and *Rickettsia conorii* in a rabbit model. Am J Trop Med Hyg 2006;74:521-525.

17. Houhamdi L, Fournier PE, Fang R, Raoult D. An experimental model of human body louse infection with *Rickettsia typhi*. Ann NY Acad Sci 2003;990:617-627.

18. Sparrow H. Infection spontanée des poux d'élevage par une rickettsia du type *Rickettsia rochalimae*. Arch Inst Pasteur Tunis 1939;28:64-73.

19. Sparrow H. Etude du foyer éthiopien de fièvre récurrente. Bull World Health Org 1958;19:673-710.

20. Houhamdi L, Raoult D. Excretion of living *Borrelia recurrentis* in feces of infected human body lice. J Infect Dis 2005;191:1898-1906.

21. Houhamdi L, Lepidi H, Drancourt M, Raoult D. Experimental model to evaluate the human body louse as a vector of plague. J Infect Dis 2006;194:1589-1596.

22. La Scola B, Raoult D. *Acinetobacter baumannii* in human body louse. Emerg Inf Dis 2004;10:1671.

23. Houhamdi L, Raoult D. Experimental infection of human body lice with Acinetobacter baumannii. Am J Trop Med Hyg 2006;74:526-531.

24. Meinking TL. Infestations. Curr Probl Dermatol 1999;11:73-120.

Internet Resources for Head Lice

12. Internet Resources for Head Lice

There is a wealth of information on the web about head lice, but much of it is non-authoritative and contains inaccurate or non-original material. Medical, health and university websites abound on the internet, and many of them display head lice information. Unfortunately, most of them obtain their so-called facts with little discretion from a wide range of sources which results in them providing inaccurate, misleading and myth-based information. None are listed here because all of the sites surveyed contained misleading errors or gross omissions.

For instance, a good number of university websites from the USA in particular insist on advising people to vacuum, treat, wash and clean clothes, beds, mattresses, furniture, head gear and even cars. Any website that offers this sort of advice cannot be trusted because this advice is based on old myths and is not evidence-based. As a consequence, the following list is brief, but reliable:

Vector Control and Repellent Research Group, School of Public Health, Tropical Medicine and Rehabilitation Sciences, James Cook University (Australia)

■ DeLouse

An interactive website for the diagnosis and treatment of head lice infestations.

http://www.jcu.edu.au/school/sphtm/antonbreinl/centers/vcrrc/hl/DeLOUSE/index.htm

■ Head lice information sheet

http://www.jcu.edu.au/school/phtm/PHTM/hlice/hlinfo1.htm

■ Anatomy of head lice

- Anatomy of adult head lice

http://www.jcu.edu.au/school/phtm/PHTM/poster/lousypst.htm

- Eggs of head lice

http://www.jcu.edu.au/school/phtm/PHTM/hlice/eggs.htm

■ Biology of Head Lice

- An excellent lecture on the biology of head lice

http://www.jcu.edu.au/school/phtm/PHTM/hlice/hlbio/hlb1.htm

- How much blood do head lice drink? An interactive calculator

http://www.jcu.edu.au/school/phtm/PHTM/hlice/blood-feed-calculator.htm

■ Presentations

- Transmission of head lice, *Pediculus capitis*, and its prevention

http://www.jcu.edu.au/school/sphtm/antonbreinl/centers/vcrrc/headlicetransmission01.pdf

- Observations of stasis in head lice as a survival technique against pediculicides

http://www.jcu.edu.au/school/sphtm/antonbreinl/centers/vcrrc/licestasisposter.pdf

- The effectiveness (or failure to be precise) of DEET and botanical repellents against head lice

http://www.jcu.edu.au/school/sphtm/antonbreinl/centers/vcrrc/licerepelposter.pdf

Harvard School of Public Health: Head lice information (USA)

An excellent site with data on therapy and insecticide resistance. Includes a submission form to allow people to have specimens identified.

http://www.hsph.harvard.edu/headlice.html

National Pediculosis Association (USA)

NPA is the premier organisation involved in head lice control in the USA. The site contains a range of data on biology, treatment and control. Information is updated frequently. NPA is particularly active in promoting the "no nit policy" and physical treatments for pediculosis.

http://www.headlice.org/

Centers for Disease Control and Prevention —Head Lice (USA)

Information put together by the National Center for Zoonotic, Vector-borne and Enteric Diseases.

http://www.cdc.gov/lice/head/index.html

Wikipedia—Head Louse

An informative review of head lice based on scientific literature. Most of the external links are not to be trusted.

http://en.wikipedia.org/wiki/Head_louse

International Society of Phthirapterists

News, information on meetings, new books and publications etc. Not restricted to human lice.

http://www.phthiraptera.org

Pediculosis.com

A website sponsored by Albyn Limited, a producer of head lice combs. Up-to-date information on ongoing studies, media feedback and publications. Focus on the head lice industry.

http://www.pediculosis.com

Susan and Steve Seale's: All you never wanted to know about head lice

A very practical site that addresses a very broad range of issues on pediculosis. Includes some good scanning electron micrographs of *Pediculus capitis* and eggs. The section analysing alternative treatments is outstanding.

http://home.hiwaay.net/~sseale/ftest.html

Virtual Parenting—Head lice video

This video describes and demonstrates the techniques on the head lice information sheet.

http://www.virtualparenting.com.au/

Lice Mare

A hi-tech personal account of pediculosis from Micscape Magazine (http://www.microscopy-uk.org.uk/mag/indexmag.html). This is not really an authoritative source, but has good images and excellent entertainment value!

http://www.micscape.simplenet.com/mag/art98/night4.html

A few louse-specific reference lists and bibliographies can be found on the web

- Copies of papers authored and co-authored by Professor Rick Speare

http://www.jcu.edu.au/school/phtm/PHTM/hlice/hladd.htm

- Bibliography of lice parasitic on humans

http://www.jcu.edu.au/school/phtm/PHTM/hlice/hlrefs.htm

- Phthiraptera Central—a reference list focussing on lice in general

http://www.refworks.com/refshare/?site=01002978336000000/459970/218471129329111000

Index

Index

A
albendazole 84
aliphatic lactones 89
area repellents 90

B
bacillary angiomatosis 132
body (clothing) louse 24

C
carbamates 57
carbaryl 58
cinnamon 80
clove 79
coconut 80
combing 48
combs 54
control of head lice
    in developed market economies 116
    in resource-poor communities 120
co-trimoxazole 84
crab louse 24
crotamiton 58
custard apple 79

D
DDT 57
DEET 89
diagnosis 48
dimeticone 73

E
eggs 27
endocarditis 132
endosymbionts of head lice 93
essential oils 88
eucalyptus 80

F
feeding 27

H
head louse 24
health education 116
home remedies 76

I
immunisation 95
incidence 41
information leaflets 117
insecticides
    chemical 56
    natural 76
itching 44
ivermectin 83

K
kdr allele frequencies 69
knockdown resistance gene mutations 66
knowledge 104, 112

L
levamisole 85
lice combs 54
lice eczema 45
life cycle 29, 30
lindane 57
Lippia species 79
louse-borne epidemic typhus 133
louse-borne relapsing fever 132, 134
lymphadenopathy 45

M
malathion 57, 58
mating 27
medical devices 124
medicinal products 126
migration routes 19
morphology 25

N
N,N-Diethyl-meta-toluamide (DEET) 89
neem 78
No Nit Policy 118
nutmeg 80
nymphs 30

O
organophosphates 57
Ovicides 80
Oxyphthirine® 87

P
peppermint 80
phenylbutazon 85
phylogenetic tree 18
phytochemicals 88
Polish plait 20
practices 107
prevalence 40
prevention 116
pubic louse 24
pyrethrins 57, 58, 77
pyrethroids 57, 58

Q
Quantitative Sequencing 67
quassia 78

R
rapid assessment method 51
Real-time PCR Amplification of Specific Allele 68
repellents 87